D1318019

Electromagn␣␣
and Your He␣␣

612   Milburn, Michael Peter.
.01442   Electromagnetic fields and your health / Michael
Mil   Milburn and Maren Oelbermann. -- Vancouver : New
         Star Books, 1994.
           xii, 207 p. : ill.

         Includes bibliographical references and index.
         06935818   ISBN 0921586302 (pbk.)

         1. Electromagnetic fields - Health aspects. 2.
         Electromagnetic fields - Safety measures. I.
         Oelbermann, Maren, 1968- II. Title

  6767   94JUN22

Electromagnetic Fields and Your Health

Michael Milburn and Maren Oelbermann

New Star Books
Vancouver
1994

Cover by Kris Klaasen / Working Design
Printed and bound in Canada by Best Gagné Book Manufacturers
1 2 3 4 5   98 97 96 95 94
First printing, May 1994

Publication of this book is made possible by grants from the Canada Council, the Department of Heritage Book Publishing Industry Development Program, and the Cultural Services Branch, Province of British Columbia

New Star Books Ltd.
2504 York Avenue
Vancouver, B.C.
V6K 1E3

Canadian Cataloguing in Publication Data

Milburn, Michael Peter.
  Electromagnetic fields and your health

  Includes bibliographical references and index.
  ISBN 0-921586-30-2

  1. Electromagnetic fields — Health aspects.   2. Electromagnetic fields — Safety measures.   I. Oelbermann, Maren, 1968-   II. Title.
RA569.3.M56 1994   612'.01442   C94-910281-4

CONTENTS

PREFACE

The twentieth century has given rise to monumental changes in the way we live. People have been taken from the horse and buggy to the moon. By the 1950s the sense of optimism about technology was overflowing, and the rush was on to take advantage of the new conveniences afforded by mass production and a frenzy of invention. There seemed no limit to progress.

Perhaps Rachel Carson's book *Silent Spring* was the pin that burst our optimism about the expanding balloon of technology. The fact that technological progress often comes at a high price could no longer be ignored. The damage to the environment from pesticides — the subject of Carson's book — has proved to be the tip of an iceberg. A scrutiny of human activities on the planet has pointed to effects that seem to threaten even the basic ecosystems upon which all life depends.

Electricity has not escaped this scrutiny unscathed. We have learned more about the environmental effects of nuclear power stations, and even if you ignore Three Mile Island and Chernobyl, it is now clear that this method of power generation does not fulfill the boasts of those who hailed it as a source of power "too cheap to meter." Meanwhile, the environmental consequences of large-scale hydro development are beginning to be better understood, pointing to long-term costs that could not have been predicted at the time of construction. The connection between fossil fuel power generation and global warming, acid rain, and weakened lungs in children are being demonstrated by scientists, and even accepted by politicians. As part of this shift from technology worship to environmental concern, another curious side-effect of electricity has started to gain attention.

During the past few decades there has been an undercurrent of scientific research examining the possibility that weak electromagnetic energy fields may be able to produce changes in cells and organisms. This is the same kind of electromagnetism that surrounds common household electrical devices like hair dryers and electric blankets. It is also created by the transmission of electricity through power lines. Hundreds of research papers have now been published worldwide describing this exciting new area of study. Ongoing scientific meetings are providing a forum for discussions of the latest developments.

While many more years of study will be required to fully understand this complex subject, it is quickly becoming an established area of research. Some scientists feel that continued study may provide new insights into our understanding of living things. This research has created intense debate in the scientific community, since many of the observations have no apparent explanation. At the same time, a question has been raised: if the kind of electromagnetism associated with power lines and electrical devices is able to affect cells and tissues, could there be an association between these electromagnetic fields and human health? It is this question which has caught public attention.

Members of the public have become aware that there is a worldwide research effort surrounding the question of human health effects from low-frequency magnetic fields. Workers in so-called electrical occupations are being studied to see if they are at an increased risk of a number of life-threatening illnesses. A number of lawsuits from police officers whose cancers may be related to the microwaves from radar guns are now working their way through the legal system. The courts have had to consider whether power lines adjacent to school property pose a threat to children's safety, and rule on cases dealing with depression of real estate values due to power lines. These examples il-lustrate that the scientific debate is now accompanied by an emotionally charged controversy in the public domain.

The background to this issue has not been clearly presented to the public. The mass media tend to focus on crisis situations, and their stories generally lack depth. Meanwhile, the scientific review bodies are sifting the research studies carried out to date and are attempting to draw some definite conclusions with re-spect to the implications for human health. They are faced with many conflicting scientific opinions. Many members of the pub-lic are confused about whether they should be concerned.

The reason for this confusion can be illustrated by a recent media report. This wire service story noted that a major media union, the Newspaper Guild, recommended that its members re-strict their use of cellular phones. The article also mentioned a lawsuit by a Florida man alleging that cellular phone use played a role in his wife's death from brain cancer. The piece ended with the statement that cellular phones have been tested and de-clared safe by industry officials and health department scientists.

Such a contradictory message provides more questions than answers. Why is there an assumption of safety on the part of authorities? On what basis would people outside the scientific community demonstrate concerns and make conjectures regard-ing adverse effects on human health from electromagnetic tech-nologies? This book presents the background needed to understand the different dimensions of these questions.

A major focus of this book is the scientific debate about the interaction of weak electromagnetic fields with biological sys-tems. Fundamental questions of this type underlie the more spe-cific concerns about human health. Although there is a new scientific discipline emerging based on the study of weak energy field bioeffects, there is also an element within scientific circles that is confident on theoretical grounds of the impossibility of effects from weak fields. This has created an emotionally charged conflict between bioelectromagnetics scientists, excited about the exploration of a new frontier, and a number of powerful mainstream scientists adamantly denying even the possibility of the observations their opponents describe. This book will provide some insight into this scientific battle royal. One cannot understand the controversy over the question of health effects from electromagnetic technologies without some feeling for these basic disagreements.

Bioelectromagnetics comprises only one area of research into the relationship between electromagnetism and biology. The question of adverse health effects from electromagnetic technologies falls within the domain of another specialized discipline, epidemiology. Epidemiological studies of environmental electromagnetic fields directly address human health issues and have their own attendant controversy. Epidemiological evidence of weak field radiation effects can be dismissed by many scientists because the theoretical basis for explaining such observances have not been established. Thus, environmental electromagnetic field epidemiology and bioelectromagnetics are closely linked.

Through a discussion of the scientific studies that have been carried out, we hope to provide you with some insight into the specific technical issues being debated by researchers in the field. This is a complex and multidisciplinary subject that has been a challenge to write about, and may sometimes be a challenge to read. In order to help you find your way through the sometimes murky world of technical jargon we have included a glossary (see page 190).

After reading about the research in this area, you will no doubt agree that it is hard to dispute that these fields can affect living things, even if scientists don't know how this happens. You might also find it hard to avoid coming to the conclusion that our health is being affected to some extent by our use of electromagnetic technologies. Despite the fact that risks are not 100 per cent certain and precisely defined from a scientific perspective, it is not surprising that this issue has become very public. Perhaps the ominous and visible high voltage lines account for the strong concern over power line electromagnetic fields, but a number of other technologies — computer monitors, electric blankets and cellular telephones to name a few — have also become the subject of concern.

The first two stages in learning to live with the risks from our technologies — discovering and clearly defining the risks and studying the methods and costs of reducing these risks — are both currently the focus of attention all over the world. The third and final stage, deciding what actually to do, usually involves lowering the risks to "acceptable" levels. This process of defining what is acceptable involves human and social values, and in a democratic society demands public input. It is hoped that this book will facilitate such public involvement.

While the task of improving our understanding of weak field effects continues in concert with the very political process of deciding what to do about the risks, you may want to do something about these risks at a personal level. This is addressed in Chapter 6, where we describe some simple steps you can take to reduce your exposure to these fields that are becoming the focus of so much controversy. The strategy of "prudent avoidance" — reducing contact with fields by using simple and cost-effective steps — strikes a balance between the need for electromagnetic technology and a desire to minimize any personal risk.

Those parts of this book dealing with basic questions about the interaction of weak energy fields and living organisms have been written as a result of the work of scientists who have put their energy and enthusiasm wholeheartedly into the exploration of the frontiers of scientific knowledge. These men and women have not been afraid to tackle the tough questions that should be asked. It is because of their efforts that a book such as this can be written. Special thanks to those scientists who kindly provided extensive information on their research. Those members of the public who have developed an open-minded sense of inquiry and maintain an interest in complex subjects such as the topic of this book have been a major source of inspiration to the authors.

There are many individuals who helped in one way or another to make this book possible. We are especially grateful for their assistance. Special thanks to Doug Milburn and Wey Herng Leong for help with graphics, Chris Milburn for his help with research, and Mike Sr. and Inga Milburn for their criticism of the manuscript. Our publisher and editor Rolf Maurer deserves special mention for his belief in this project. Without his support this book would have never been more than a good idea.

Electromagnetic Fields and Your Health

ONE

INTRODUCTION

In 1990, a United States Environmental Protection Agency (EPA) draft report classified low-frequency magnetic fields as Class B carcinogens, a class reserved for substances considered as "probable human carcinogens." This would compare such fields to PCBs, formaldehyde and DDT. Considering that low-frequency magnetic fields are ubiquitous features of our modern lifestyle, it is hard to imagine that hair dryers, electric blankets and power lines would produce something that demands such a frightening comparison. Although this EPA report was criticized and later revised to remove low-frequency magnetic fields from classification, such an incident only served to increase public concern and highlight the controversy within the scientific community.

There are several basic elements to the scientific controversy. Firstly, there is the fundamental question of whether weak electromagnetic energy fields are able to cause changes in living things. Some scientists feel there are theoretical reasons why these weak fields should not cause biological effects. However, the many observations actually demonstrating biological changes from weak electromagnetic fields give rise to the second controversial question: how in fact could these changes come about if they were not supposed to happen in the first place? There is an emotionally charged debate currently going on among scientists who, on one extreme, feel that the study of electromagnetic field bioeffects is a most important scientific frontier, and on the other feel that these fields could not possibly influence living systems. It is an exciting time for scientists when new and unexpected results emerge.

A separate, but intimately connected issue arises from this debate. The biological activity of weak electromagnetic energy fields has suggested to epidemiologists, those scientists interested in the many factors associated with human disease, that these "weak" fields should be studied for a possible connection to human health. If the types of exposures incurred by living near a power line, using an electric blanket or working as a welder are able to produce changes in our cells and tissues, they may be able to affect our health. The debate surrounding this issue is even more heated than in the case of the basic questions about how weak fields can produce biological changes of any kind. The controversial nature of each new epidemiological study is assured even before its completion because of the potential far-reaching consequences of its results and conclusions. This book will explore all these areas that comprise what is fast becoming one of the most talked about issues of the 1990s.

BIOELECTROMAGNETICS: A NEW SCIENTIFIC FRONTIER

Powerful electromagnetic waves such as X-rays can be very harmful to living organisms. The biological effects of X-rays and other forms of so-called ionizing radiation have been studied for some time. However, the relationship between much less powerful non-ionizing electromagnetic radiation and living systems is also now being investigated. Non-ionizing electromagnetic radiation includes the kinds of fields produced by power lines, hair dryers and electric blankets. Some aspects of these investigations have become known as bioelectromagnetics. In the words of one bioelectromagnetics researcher:

In the recent past, research was almost exclusively motivated by the need to better understand [weak electromagnetic fields] as possible harmful environmental agents. However, it is also becoming increasingly clear that biological [weak electromagnetic field] interactions deserve to be studied in their own right, as there is increasing evidence that low intensity electromagnetic energy interactions might be fundamental to life processes. Furthermore, the potential therapeutic use of [weak electromagnetic fields] also seems to be promising. First, however, scientists need to understand the mechanistic basis of biological weak field interactions before [electromagnetic field] treatment protocols can be designed on a rational basis. The discipline devoted to the study of the above research issue is called "bioelectromagnetics".[1]

An interaction between weak electromagnetic energy fields and living organisms is not predicted on the basis of current scientific thinking, and thus the observation of effects at very low electromagnetic field levels constitutes a scientific frontier. One of the most controversial and challenging periods of scientific inquiry occurs when observations are made that are not easily explainable in terms of current theories.

Over the past few decades, bioelectromagnetics scientists have examined a wide range of phenomena. They have studied the effects of magnetic fields on the daily rhythmic cycles in animals ranging from oysters and rats to man. Bioelectromagnetics scientists have found a magnetic navigational sense in pigeons and have studied the changes in the proteins produced by a cell's DNA as a result of electromagnetic field exposure. They have observed electromagnetic field-induced changes in cells that are important in the function of the immune system. Magnetic crystals have been found in the human brain. By using weak electromagnetic fields, scientists are studying the communication between cells. Though it is a little-known discipline, even among scientists, bioelectromagnetics has become a broad area of scientific investigation.

Scientific inquiry by its very nature is a conservative enterprise and does not easily have its basic paradigm challenged. As biological effects from weak electromagnetic energy fields are not supposed to exist at all, a scientific battle royal is under way as the different personalities within scientific circles conflict. This is a side of science not often seen by the public.

Bioelectromagnetics scientists have often expressed a sense of frustration at the lack of acceptance of their research. In some cases, they have noted the words of scientists involved in past frontier developments. For example, the famous physicist Max Planck, well acquainted with controversy in his key role in the revolutionary quantum theory at the turn of the century, remarked on changes in scientific ideas:

> *An important scientific innovation rarely makes its way by gradually winning over its opponents: it rarely happens that Saul becomes Paul. What does happen is that its opponents gradually die out and that the growing generation is familiarized with the idea from the beginning.*[2]

Science develops ideas within the framework of particular models, and the assumptions of these models are not challenged without controversy. Perhaps this is not so different from other areas of society when dealing with change. As the 19th century philosopher William James said:

> *When a thing is new people said — "It is not true." Later, when its truth became obvious, people said — "Anyway, it is not important." And when its importance could not be denied, people said — "Anyway, it is not new."*[3]

Much of the new bioelectromagnetics research has remained obscure despite the exciting possibility of important new developments in our understanding of biological systems, and the significant potential for new medical techniques arising out of the new knowledge. New developments in medicine based on exploring the relationship between electromagnetism and biology include using pulsed magnetic fields to promote the healing of bones, and new cancer treatments developed by the Swedish radiologist Björn Nordenström based on his ideas of what he calls biologically closed electric circuits. However, the separate yet related epidemiological investigation of man-made weak fields and their relationship to human health has brought the study of the interaction between living organisms and electromagnetic fields out of obscurity and into the limelight.

NATURAL ELECTROMAGNETIC ENERGY FIELDS

Before a discussion of the many electromagnetic fields created by our use of electromagnetic technologies, it is useful to examine our natural exposure to electromagnetic energy fields. The earth produces a magnetic field which ranges from 350 to 700 milligauss (mG) over the surface of the planet. This is a static (direct current, or DC) field which can be visualized as a bar magnet inside the earth with a south and a north pole. There are many variations in the geomagnetic field corresponding to daily and yearly rhythms as well as various sunspot cycles. An electric field is also present at the earth's surface which shows large changes with the weather. This electric field is associated with charge differences between the earth and the atmosphere.

Lightning helps to activate so-called Schumann resonances and produces electromagnetic waves ranging from low frequency to radio frequencies which propagate over long distances. The earth and the ionosphere form a resonant cavity where low-frequency electromagnetic waves can propagate. The

Schumann resonances produce low-frequency electromagnetic waves with a maximum strength at around 10 cycles per second (Hz). Natural low-frequency magnetic fields are very weak and can range from 0.001 mG around 5 Hz to less than 0.0000001 mG over 100 Hz. Of course, visible light is one of the most important types of electromagnetic energy found at the earth's surface. Very low levels of other types of electromagnetic energy, such as X-rays and radio waves, are also present.

The more obvious interactions of these natural forms of electromagnetic energy with life on the planet include our visual sense and photosynthesis in plants, both of which make use of visible electromagnetic energy. Interactions of low-frequency magnetic fields (including DC) with living things are one of the areas of bioelectromagnetics research.[4] Bacteria have been found with small crystals of magnetite for sensing magnetic fields. These magnetotactic organisms have a built-in compass and make use of the earth's geomagnetic field.[5] Pigeons, bees and some mammals also have been found to have a magnetic navigational capability.[6] In fact, researchers have recently discovered magnetic crystals in the human brain. Perhaps humans also once utilized the earth's magnetism for navigation with their own on-board compass — or we still rely on it in ways we don't know about.

The circadian rhythms of humans have been shown to have a sensitivity to very weak low-frequency electromagnetic fields.[7] In experiments where human subjects lived in underground rooms, the German scientist Rütger Wever showed that when shielded from the earth's magnetic field there was a desynchronization in the subjects' internal rhythms. More interestingly, the circadian rhythm could be restored by application of a very weak electric field at a frequency of 10 Hz. It has even been suggested that natural electromagnetic fields may have played a role in the origin of life itself.[8] A number of authors[9] suggest that although exposure to natural electromagnetic fields is limited, organisms may be sensitive to these fields.

Such ideas are not new. In a book entitled *Electromagnetic*

Fields and Life,[10] first published in 1968, the Russian scientist A.S. Presman discusses the interaction of weak electromagnetic energy fields with living systems. Through detailed examination of the many studies already carried out in both the former Soviet Union and the West by that time, Presman put forward a hypothesis that electromagnetic energy is important for the transfer of information. He postulated that electromagnetic energy may be used by the organism to gain information from the environment,[11] that it plays a role in organization and control within the organism,[12] and that it may even be used for communication between organisms.[13]

Work on this frontier has continued despite a lack of support from mainstream science, which is more focused on the biochemical aspects of biology. For example, in his introduction to a fascinating book edited by F.A. Popp published in 1989, *Electromagnetic Bioinformation*, Dr. K.H. Li writes:

Now there is evidence that it is the informational aspect of biological systems that characterizes the essential view of life. And this is less reflected by biochemical findings but rather by a level beyond the domain of chemical reactivity, namely that of electromagnetic fields. Within the framework of electromagnetic bioinformation a basic explanation of biological processes eg. communication, health, ageing, cancer, biological rhythms, regulation and biochemical control may be found and not just their description. At the same time the interrelation between all these different phenomenon becomes evident.[14]

It is difficult to explain, using the biochemical paradigm that dominates the biological sciences today, how weak electromagnetic energy fields could directly affect living organisms. This is but one reason why some scientists have begun to challenge this paradigm; the result of this challenge may be a new way of understanding living things.[15]

POLLUTION FROM ELECTRICITY?

Only time will tell to what extent such radical new ideas will further our knowledge of living things. In any case, such developments may not be necessary to establish a better understanding of electromagnetic energy bioeffects, and the relationship of exposures to weak fields from sources such as electric blankets or power lines to human health. There already exist a number of proposed mechanisms for electromagnetic energy bioeffects, and the number of epidemiological studies is increasing. These studies will help us evaluate the relationship between human health and the man-made changes in our electromagnetic environment. Chapters 3 and 4 examine the basic scientific elements of this controversy.

Our natural electromagnetic environment has been drastically altered by technology over the past century. It has been recognized since the 1970s that major changes in our electromagnetic environment have occurred, and the term "electromagnetic pollution" has been applied to describe man-made environmental electromagnetic energy fields. In 1974 the United States Office of Telecommunications Policy suggested that we may soon find ourselves in an "era of energy pollution comparable to that of chemical pollution today."[16]

In 1976, a book called *Electromagnetism, Man and the Environment*, by Dr. J.H. Battocletti, was published.[17] Even before the 1979 Wertheimer-Leeper paper on childhood leukemia (discussed later in this book) touched off a long series of epidemiological studies, Battocletti warned that weak electromagnetic field effects were important and that electrical pollution could be compared with the more well known forms of pollution:

> *Yes, non-thermal electrical pollution exists. More and more knowledgeable people are beginning to hold this view. Non-thermal electrical pollution is most severe when waves modulated by frequencies which coincide with biological frequencies are used. Fortunately, there are many more cases of electromagnetic*

*radiation which do not fall into this category. Much more re-
search is required to verify this conclusion, and to delineate
those types of non-thermal pollution which are to be avoided.*

*In our technological age, we cannot avoid being immersed in
a sea of electrical, magnetic and electromagnetic fields . . . We
must avoid these hazardous fields just as we must avoid harmful water, air, noise, and thermal pollution.*[17]

In 1981, the World Health Organization (WHO) expressed a
similar concern.[18] In a report in their Environmental Health series, WHO suggested that harmful side effects accompany many
beneficial technologies due to changes they create in our environment. They noted the awareness of pollution by chemicals,
noise and ionizing radiation and pointed out that exposures to
non-ionizing electromagnetic energy "now exceeds that from
natural sources," and that "the rapid proliferation of such
sources and substantial increase in radiation levels is likely to
produce 'electromagnetic pollution'."

"Electromagnetic pollution" is a ubiquitous feature of modern
life. It is 60 Hz electromagnetic energy that is most commonly
experienced. In our homes, invisible magnetic and electric fields
are present which change direction sixty times per second. These
fields are produced by nearby power lines, electrical wiring in
our homes and the many electrical devices that we routinely use.
Additionally, communications systems, radio and television
transmitters, military radar installations and personal hobbies
expose us to myriad frequencies in the microwave and radio
wave bands. Computers, fluorescent lights and the many other
electrical devices that are fixtures of the modern office produce
electromagnetic fields. Welders, aluminium smelter and power
utility workers and others employed in so-called electrical occupations experience electromagnetic fields. Chapter 2 explores
the many ways in which we encounter fields in our daily lives.

In fact, it is hard to escape from this deluge of electromagnetic energy. Power lines trace our highway and roadway networks, electric buses and trains crisscross the countryside, and

communications systems of many types send their signals to the far corners of the globe. Things are getting so bad that electromagnetic interference between electronic and electrical equipment is now a major problem; scientists using radio telescopes to observe the weak radio signals emitted by many astronomical bodies are complaining that electromagnetic "smog" is greatly hindering their work.

The European Community is working on regulations to create strict standards for all electronic and electrical equipment in an attempt to limit electromagnetic interference between electromagnetic technologies. This will even apply to electronic children's toys. Ironically, researchers testing for electromagnetic interference are having great difficulty in finding a non-polluted environment in which they can test new devices with precision; an English company was forced to use an underground salt mine. Will there soon be *any* electromagnetic pollution-free environments to be found?[19]

'ONE OF THE MOST TALKED ABOUT HEALTH ISSUES OF THE 1990s'

What is the effect on our health and well-being from these changes to our natural electromagnetic environment? As scientists around the globe attempt to answer this question, the public dimensions of this controversial issue are expanding. News headlines appear regularly, and every year more lawsuits relating to electrical pollution are launched. As one information booklet used by power utilities states, the electromagnetic field issue "promises to be one of the most talked-about health issues of the 1990's."

There are both personal and public dimensions to any health issue. From a personal perspective, our responses depend on our definition of health. A broad definition has been put forth by the World Health Organization.[20] From this perspective, if electromagnetic energy fields are found to be related to health effects such as reduced immune system responses, behavioural changes, or depression, this is cause for concern. From a public health perspective, significant increases in life-threatening diseases have to be well established before authorities will act. It should be emphasised that public health considerations do not provide the kind of blanket assurances of safety the public often seems to expect. From a public health perspective, what is "safe" is a question of risk/benefit analysis. That is, some risks are associated with many (if not all) technological developments and human activities, and these risks are to be evaluated in relation to the benefits of the new technologies. This involves the concept of acceptable risk, something which unconsciously is part of the many decisions made daily in our lives. At the broader social level, it is important that the individuals most affected are part of the decision-making process to define what is acceptable. Chapter 5 discusses the public dimensions of this issue.

Increasingly, researchers are examining the issue of risks from weak electromagnetic energy fields. It is a difficult problem to separate the many risk factors for human diseases, and more research is required for this relatively new field of scientific endeavour. (The current state of epidemiological research is discussed in Chapter 3.) Without the kind of precise data on health and the consensus of scientists that the public health apparatus requires, individuals are left to consider environmental electromagnetic fields from a personal perspective. One approach suggested to date is to practice what has been called "prudent avoidance". This is discussed in Chapter 6.

While statistical studies of the health of large populations are still under way, personal stories of the possible impact of electromagnetic energy field exposure are beginning to appear in the media. For example, a 1991 *Harrowsmith* article on this issue[21] featured the story of a 6-year-old suffering from leukemia whose family lived in the countryside near Toronto. After their son was diagnosed with leukemia, the boy's oncologist provided the parents with information about electromagnetic fields. Measurements in the boy's bedroom revealed that his bed was located in

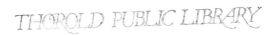

an area of higher-than-average low-frequency magnetic fields from the household wiring. The boy's mother was not sure that this was related to her son's illness, but took the precaution of moving the bed to an area of the bedroom with lower fields. The family has since taken steps to reduce their exposure to other sources of electromagnetic fields in their home.

A 1991 story in the newsletter *Microwave News*[22] was part of a series of articles on cancer concerns from the use of police radar units. This feature discussed a number of lawsuits from police officers alleging their cancers were related to the use of radar while on traffic duty. One officer, whose radar unit was mounted in his cruiser just behind his head, developed a melanoma on the back of his neck. The cancers of two Californian officers were reported to have occurred at the places where they rested their radar guns; one officer developed a lymphoma in his groin, and the other developed a lymphoma on his leg.

Some scientists regard such anecdotal reports as media sensationalism which does nothing to assist in the effort to understand better the relationship between weak fields and human health. Members of the public, however, are generally not too impressed by statistical data reporting "proportional mortality ratios" and "confidence intervals". Stories of actual people and tragedy get attention, and many individuals seem to be sceptical of scientific data, pointing to the possible sources of influence on the conclusions. This gap represents one of the many misunderstandings and sources of frustration between scientific authorities and the public. In the following chapters we examine further the different aspects of this issue.

CHAPTER 1 NOTES

1. Walleczek, J. (1992) "The Immune System and ELF Electromagnetic Fields." *Frontier Perspectives*, 3:1.

2. Planck, M.K.E.L. (1932) *Where is Science Going?* New York: Norton.

3. James, W. Quoted in Fröhlich, Herbert (1988) *Biological Coherence and Response to External Stimuli*. Berlin: Springer Verlag.

4. The reader is referred to the following sources for more information on this topic:
Smith, C.W. and S. Best (1989) *Electromagnetic Man*. New York: St. Martin's Press.
Persinger, M.A. (1974) *ELF and VLF Electromagnetic Field Effects*. New York: Plenum Press.

5. See for example: Polk, C. and E. Postow (1986) *CRC Handbook of Biological Effects of Electromagnetic Fields*. Florida: CRC Press.

6. For further reading see: Becker, R.O. (1990) *Cross Currents: The Promise of Electromagnetism, the Perils of Electropollution*. Los Angeles: Jeremy P. Tarcher Inc.

7. Wever, R. (1974) "ELF Effects on Human Circadian Rhythms." In Persinger, M.A. *ELF and VLF Electromagnetic Field Effects*. New York: Plenum Press, 101-144.

8. Cole, F.E. and E.R. Graf (1974) "Precambrian ELF and Abiogenesis." In Persinger, M.A. *ELF and VLF Electromagnetic Field Effects*. New York: Plenum Press, 243-275.

9. A number of authors suggest that biological organisms are sensitive to electromagnetic fields. See for example:
Presman, A.S. (1970) *Electromagnetic Fields and Life*. New York: Plenum Press.
Smith, C.W. and S. Best (1989) *Electromagnetic Man*. New York: St. Martin's Press.
Popp, F.A. *et al.*, eds. (1989) *Electromagnetic Bioinformation*, Second edition. Munich: Urban und Schwarzenberg.

10. The English translation of *Electromagnetic Fields and Life* was published in 1970 by Plenum Press and translated by F.L. Sinclair. Presman, A.S. (1970) *Electromagnetic Fields and Life*. New York: Plenum Press.

11. Examples of this include bacteria, bees and pigeons sensing the earth's magnetic field for use in navigation. Experiments by Wever suggest that the low-frequency component of the earth's magnetic field may be a *Zeitgeber* (time giver) for human circadian rhythms.

12. Some frontier researchers suggest that electromagnetic energy systems yet undiscovered may be important features of life in addition to the nervous system. Could the meridians used in acupuncture be re-

lated to this concept, as they seem to represent some sort of internal energy system for communications control?

13. For example, sharks are able to sense the very low electrical fields of their prey. In fact, they are known to damage undersea telecommunication cables, apparently mistaking the electromagnetic fields of the cables for those of live fish.

Another interesting example is the experiments on termites by Günther Becker, published in Popp, F.A., ed. (1989) *Electromagnetic Bioinformation*, Second edition. Munich: Urban und Schwarzenberg, 116. Becker postulates a non-chemical information system within the termite colony and suggests that the biofields of the termites were sensed by other termites.

14. Popp, F.A. (1989) *Electromagnetic Bioinformation*. Munich: Urban und Schwarzenberg.

15. As Presman pointed out in *Electromagnetic Fields and Life*, the use of electromagnetic energy by biological systems may occur at the level of the organism as a whole and may not be evident at molecular levels. The discoveries of modern biology have used a reductionist methodology whereby the workings of the inner biochemical machinery have been scrutinized. Perhaps there is a basic conflict in approach, that is, in the prior assumptions underlying scientific inquiry that need to be overcome in bioelectromagnetics. The need for a more holistic approach in biology and medicine has been discussed by others. For example see Capra, F. (1982) *The Turning Point*. New York: Simon and Schuster.

16. *Electromagnetics News* (1991) 2:2-3.

17. Battocletti, J.H. (1976) *Electromagnetism, Man and the Environment*. London: Elek Books.

18. World Health Organization (1981) *Environmental Health Criteria 16, Radiofrequency and Microwaves*. Geneva.

19. *Electromagnetics News* (1991) 2:4-5.

20. The WHO's definition of health: "Health is a state of complete physical, mental and social well-being and not merely the absence of disease or infirmity."

21. Scanlan, L. (1991) "The Killing Fields." *Harrowsmith Magazine* January/February.

22. *Microwave News* (1991) 11:2.

TWO

THE ELECTROMAGNETIC
FIELDS AROUND US

The development of technologies that use electricity and electromagnetic waves has progressed steadily over the past century.
This development has transformed the way we live our lives in
the modern world. Electric lights, television, radio and electric
stoves are but a few of the technologies that would now be considered basic necessities of life.

After the Second World War, radar and other radio and microwave technologies were introduced at a rapid pace. The heating
ability of these electromagnetic waves was recognized, and after
microwave heating effects were better understood this technology
made its way into our homes in the form of microwave ovens. It
was also recognized that humans should be protected from heating levels of radio and microwaves, and appropriate safety guidelines for high intensity electromagnetic energy were designed.

However, microwaves and radio waves, at levels below that required to produce heating, were not considered to have any biological effect. Electromagnetic energy fields with even less
energy than microwaves and radio waves, like the 60 Hz fields
produced by our home's electrical systems, were also assumed to
have no ability to affect living organisms. Thus, for the past century, the development of electric and electromagnetic technol-

ogy has occurred in the context of an underlying assumption that the associated electromagnetic energy fields could not interact with our cells and tissues or be responsible for changes in human health. In light of the present controversy over the observations that electromagnetic energy can affect biological activity at levels below that required to cause heating, it is of interest to consider what kinds of exposures are experienced in our daily lives.

ELECTROMAGNETIC FIELDS IN THE WORKPLACE

Many occupations are associated with exposure to weak electromagnetic energy. Electric arc welding, for example, creates magnetic fields that are significantly above typical background levels. Power utility working environments will result in higher than average exposure to 60 Hz magnetic and electric fields. Within the power utility organization there are many different jobs, each of which will have a unique exposure pattern (see Figure 1). Airline pilots experience electromagnetic energy from the airplane's electrical systems in the cockpit, electronics, radar and communication systems.

Microwave radar is used by police officers to monitor traffic speed. Aluminium workers are exposed to very high magnetic fields in the potrooms where the refining of aluminium takes place. These fields are created by the large DC currents that are needed to extract the aluminium from the bauxite.[1]

The modern office environment also provides opportunity for exposure to weak electromagnetic fields. The use of computers and their associated video display terminals (VDTs) is now widespread both in the office and in the home. In the VDT, a cathode-ray tube takes a beam of electrons and shoots it onto a screen, and the screen lights up where it is struck by the electron beam. Many different electronic circuits are required to accelerate an electron beam and move it around to produce an image on the screen. Magnetic fields with frequencies ranging from 50

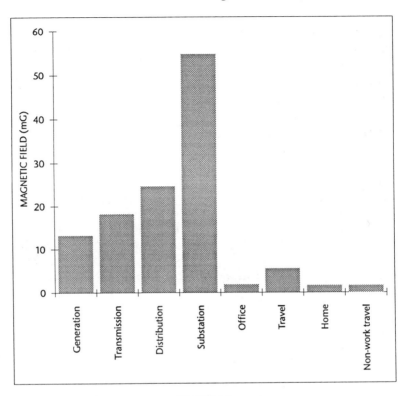

FIGURE 1
Average (arithmetic mean) magnetic fields encountered in different utility working environments as measured by an EMDEX. Many utility jobs
have higher exposures than other occupations. Adapted from data in
the 1991 NIOSH report: *Proceedings of the Scientific Workshop on the
Health Effects of Electric and Magnetic Fields on Workers.*

to 80 Hz are produced by circuits that move the electron beam
up and down. Fields with frequencies from 15,000 to 85,000 Hz
are created by the circuits moving the beam back and forth.
Magnetic fields at other frequencies will also be present, including the 60 Hz power frequency. A VDT is also surrounded by
electric fields with a range of frequencies. The computer operator sits in close proximity to the unit and thus will be exposed to

electromagnetic fields produced by the VDT's electronic circuits. As will be discussed in more detail in Chapter 5, guidelines on the electromagnetic fields from VDTs have been introduced in Sweden.

ELECTROMAGNETIC FIELDS IN THE HOME

Now let us examine the situation at home by considering two types of possible sources of weak electromagnetic energy. (Keep in mind that "weak" means non-thermal and non-ionizing — terms explained in Chapter 4 — and does not imply that these fields have no biological effects.) Firstly, there will be background (ambient) fields from such things as power lines, radio broadcast stations and household wiring. Secondly, the many electrical devices used routinely in the home will produce electromagnetic fields.

There will always be a background level of electromagnetic energy. This level will typically be higher in the city than in the country. A background 60 Hz field will be present due to high voltage transmission lines, primary and secondary electrical distribution systems, power transformers, substations, and the wiring in your home. Transmission lines carry electrical energy from its source (for example, a hydroelectric generating station) to the population centres where it is needed. This high-voltage electricity is transformed into lower-voltage energy, which is then spread within the population centre through the primary distribution network. The voltage is lowered once again, and the electricity is carried to our homes by the secondary distribution system.

Electric fields from power lines are greatest near the high-voltage lines that have captured so much attention in the media. Magnetic fields, in contrast, are related to the currents in the line. (Terms like voltage and current are defined in the Glossary, page 190.) This means that a power line which looks ominous with its large, unsightly metal pylons, may have magnetic fields that are not necessarily much different from those of a high-current primary distribution line in a high-density urban neighbourhood. It is the largest *currents*, and not the *voltages*, that are related to higher magnetic fields. The magnetic fields from transformers and substations typically fall off in strength relatively quickly with distance.

Surprisingly, the wiring in our homes may also produce higher than average background magnetic fields. This can be caused by a number of different situations.[2] One phenomenon that is now gaining attention is that unbalanced ground return currents can produce higher than average magnetic fields in a home (see Figure 2). The wires in a home occur in pairs, with each carrying currents in opposite directions from the other. If some of the current in one of the wires is fed off into the grounding system of the home, the currents will not be equal. Unequal currents produce unequal magnetic fields that do not cancel each other out, hence higher than average fields will result in the home. This phenomenon is fairly complex and depends on the way the plumbing system is used to ground the electrical wires in a home. It has been observed that higher than average fields in a home, due to the unbalanced ground return current phenomenon, sometimes have their root cause in what is going on in a neighbour's home. This is because currents can flow from a neighbour's home through the common plumbing system, into your home and back to the power line (this will not happen if plastic water mains are used).

Other types of electromagnetic energy fields can be found in a home. For example, radio signals are always present; a quick tune through your radio dial will demonstrate this. The intensity of these signals will be above average only in special cases, for example, if you were to live in close proximity to a radio transmitter.[3]

There are many other possible sources of increased background radio or microwave fields. It is hard to generalize about

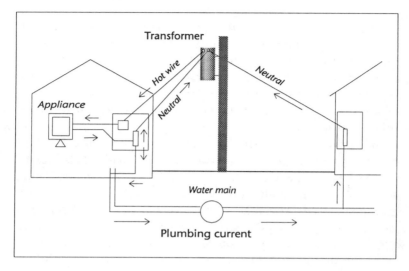

FIGURE 2
The unbalanced ground return phenomenon can sometimes be the dominant source of background magnetic fields inside a home. Instead of flowing back to the transformer through the neutral wire, some of the return current can flow into the plumbing system where it can return to the transformer through the neutral wire of a neighbour's home. Adapted from a Monitor Industries report: *Wiring Modifications to Reduce Magnetic Fields*, by Ed Leeper, March 1992.

the strength of these fields because the sources may be directional and have a wide range in their power output. The background levels experienced from radio/microwave sources will be below the safety limit designed to prevent health effects related to the heating ability of these higher frequency electromagnetic waves.

The use of electromagnetic devices will also result in increased levels of electric and magnetic fields. As shown in Table 1 on magnetic measurements, these fields decrease quickly with distance. The actual fields experienced by using a device will depend on how close you are to the device while you're using it and how far the fields extend from the device in question. Let's take a tour of the house and identify some of the more common sources of electromagnetic fields.

In the bedroom, electric blankets and waterbed heaters are two possible sources of 60 Hz magnetic fields. Motor-driven clocks (i.e., clocks with analog as opposed to LCD or LED displays) are also magnetic field sources, but high magnetic fields may only be experienced if the clock is placed within arm's reach. Magnetic fields from incandescent lights are insignificant sources, but a fluorescent bed light will produce electric and magnetic fields. Sometimes beds may be placed along a wall near where the electrical utility line enters the building, and the local magnetic fields of these wires may extend over the space where the bed has been placed.

In the bathroom, electric shavers, hair dryers and curling

TABLE 1

60 Hz MAGNETIC FIELDS* OF
VARIOUS ELECTRICAL HOUSEHOLD DEVICES

ELECTRICAL DEVICE	FIELD AT 5 CM	FIELD AT 15 CM	FIELD AT 30 CM
Toaster	5 mG	0.7 mG	0.2 mG
Electric stove	97 mG	20 mG	4 mG
Electric kettle	6 mG	2 mG	1 mG
Food processor	98 mG	30 mG	10 mG
Fluorescent light	97 mG	30 mG	10 mG
Hair dryer	>100 mG	20 mG	3 mG
Electric shaver	>100 mG	100 mG	50 mG
Refrigerator	7 mG	3 mG	1.8 mG
Television	50 mG	12 mG	5 mG

* Fields will vary depending on the model and the power level to which the device is turned.

irons are all sources of magnetic fields that are held close to the body while in use. Fluorescent lighting around a mirror will produce higher than background electric and magnetic fields.

The kitchen has one of the highest concentrations of electromagnetic technology in the home. The microwave oven creates magnetic fields, and microwaves will leak from the door seal, especially as the unit gets older. Electric stoves and ovens, refrigerators and dishwashers create magnetic fields which fall off rapidly with distance. Food processors, electric knives, electric can openers, and kettles are other common magnetic field sources in the kitchen.

In the living room, the television is one obvious source of electric and magnetic fields. Home computers and stereo systems will also add to the electric and magnetic field level. Again, whether levels of fields above background are experienced from a device will depend on how the device is used and how far the fields extend. Television use, for example, may not create higher-than-background fields because it is normal to sit at least several meters away. However, children who sit just a few feet from the television will experience an increased level of magnetic fields.

Another possible magnetic field source in the home is ceiling cable electric heat. This is rarely used, but deserves mention for the magnetic fields it can create in the home. Also, cordless and cellular telephones produce high-frequency electromagnetic waves. The cellular phone is a stronger source than the cordless phone. Hobbies such as amateur radio and CB radio, the use of electric drills and vacuum cleaners, and other commonly used electrical devices can also create exposure to above background levels of 60 Hz magnetic and electric fields as well as higher-frequency electromagnetic waves.

MEASURING THE FIELDS

Until recently little was known about many of the electromagnetic fields present in the home and workplace. Since they were not considered important biologically, few measurements of these fields had been done. Few instruments were available to effectively take low-frequency field measurements, and even now it is not well understood which features of the fields indicate potential biological consequences. Ionizing radiations such as X-rays have a well-defined measurement process and dosimetry, and X-rays can be measured in a way that is relevant to the effects of these high-energy waves on matter and people. In contrast, at this time, we really have no clear idea of what constitutes a dose of electromagnetic energy below levels that cause heating effects.

Many parameters of electromagnetic fields can be measured. Sources of low-frequency fields have both electric and magnetic components, often with one of these components dominating. Electromagnetic fields can have single or multiple frequencies and can vary over the day. Abrupt changes in fields can also be observed. Magnetic fields from electrical power lines with multiple conductors can produce quite complex fields.

The Electric Power Research Institute (EPRI), a research body funded by power utilities, has played a major role in the development of instrumentation and characterization of exposures. For example, EPRI has developed powerful computer programs to calculate fields around high-voltage transmission lines. According to EPRI:

> *Getting accurate information on the strength and distribution of these fields is crucial to the soundness of study results and, more generally, to the understanding of the baseline presence of [electromagnetic fields] in the modern environment. It is in exposure assessment that EPRI has perhaps made the most headway to date.*[4]

Probably the most significant EPRI-sponsored improvement in the ability to measure fields is the Electric and Magnetic Digital Exposure system (EMDEX). The EMDEX is a small battery-powered unit that can be worn around the waist. The lightweight instrument will take measurements of both 60 Hz magnetic and electric fields. This allows surveys of exposures in the home and workplace during a whole day or longer. The data can be analyzed by a computer using software developed for this purpose. Using this kind of new technology, surveys of low frequency fields in homes, schools, offices and in the workplace are being undertaken. EPRI has even built a test home to examine in detail the fields generated by different electrical set-ups. Of course, a major problem still exists in interpreting such complex data in a way that may be relevant to human health.

Such studies focus exclusively on the low-frequency fields associated with the 60 Hz power frequency. The larger question addressed in this book concerns the human health effects of a broader range of electromagnetic energy, including higher-frequency waves such as radio and microwaves at levels too weak to cause heating effects. These higher frequencies have not gained the same attention as the lower frequencies associated with normal household current, but with increasing use of personal devices such as cellular phones, there is more and more interest in measuring environmental levels of radio/microwaves. Up to now, radio and microwave levels have been measured for compliance with safety guidelines related to the heating ability of these waves. As safety questions over cellular phones have recently become a headline issue, interest in characterizing, in more detail, these weaker levels of the high-frequency fields will grow.

Computer systems, especially the video display terminal (VDT), produce a range of low- and slightly higher-frequency fields. Fields from computers are now being extensively measured and compared. Sweden's guidelines for VDT emissions (see Chapter 5) specify allowed values in two frequency regions. Another example of interest in measuring workplace exposures to fields other than the 60 Hz power frequency is police concern over traffic speed radar units. Extensive measurements of these units have now been carried out at the request of a number of police departments. For example, in a recent report entitled "Microwave Exposure Levels Encountered by Police Traffic Radar Operators," detailed microwave measurements of different radar models and antennae mounting systems are presented, as are means for prudently reducing exposures in the future.[5] Measurements of radio waves encountered in public situations have also been carried out. The U.S. Environmental Protection Agency, for example, has made measurements of radio frequency fields in a number of locations.[6]

The development of equipment for measuring environmental and occupational electromagnetic energy is essential to understanding the relationship between human health and exposure to these fields. Actual measurements have to be incorporated into epidemiological studies in order to overcome the weaknesses of past research. As the general levels and types of public and occupational exposures are becoming better established, laboratory research using animals and cells is able to focus on the more relevant forms of exposure. And reciprocally, as laboratory studies using cells in test tubes help to elucidate fundamental features of interaction, the interpretation of exposure data in public and occupational settings will be facilitated. As will be seen in the next chapter, there is a close connection between these different facets of research.

ELECTROMAGNETIC FIELD QUESTIONNAIRE

The following survey will help readers to gain an appreciation of the possible sources of electromagnetic fields in their daily lives. The inclusion of an electromagnetic field source in this survey does not mean that it poses a risk — not enough is known about electromagnetic fields to make any such categorical statements. The strategy of "prudent avoidance," discussed in Chapter 6, implementing strategies to reduce one's overall electromagnetic exposure, is facilitated by an understanding of the sources of electromagnetic fields that we encounter.

The numbers in parentheses indicate points for each answer. Add up all your points to determine a total score.

1. How many hours per week do you watch television?

   Less than 2 hours (0)   2 to 10 hours (2) _____
   More than 10 hours (4)
   If you sit closer than 3 meters from your television, add (2).

2. How many hours per week do you use a computer (including both at home and at work)?

   Less than 2 hours (0)   2 to 10 hours (2) _____
   More than 10 hours (4)

3. How much time do you spend per week in the kitchen using a microwave oven, electric stove or oven, and other electrical appliances such as dishwashers and food processors?

   Less than 2 hours (0)   2 to 10 hours (2) _____
   More than 10 hours (4)
   If your microwave is more than 4 years old, add (2).

4. What type of heating do you use in your home?

   Forced air, wood stove or hot water (0) _____
   Electric baseboard (2)   Ceiling cable installation (4)

5. Do you own a waterbed with heater, or an electric blanket? If not, or if you turn off the waterbed heater at night or unplug the electric blanket before retiring, skip to the next question.

How often do you use your electric blanket or waterbed?

   Rarely (0)   Weekly (3)   Almost every day (6) _____

6. How often do you use an electric heating pad?

Rarely or never (0)   *Weekly (2)*   *Almost every day (4)* _____

7. How often do you use a hair dryer, curling iron or electric shaver?

Rarely or never (0)   *Weekly (2)*   *Almost every day (4)* _____

8. Add a half point for each of the following devices if you use them several times a week.

Electric kettle	*Toaster*
Food processor	*Coffee maker*
Dishwasher	*Electric grill or wok*
Electric lawn mower	*Electric iron*
Vacuum cleaner	*Sewing machine* _____

9. How often do you use a cellular phone or CB radio?

Rarely or never (0)   *Weekly (2)*   *Almost every day (4)* _____

10. How often do you use electromagnetic devices for hobby or recreation (*e.g.* amateur radio, electric welding, electronics)?

Rarely or never (0)   *Weekly (2)*   *Almost every day (4)* _____

11. Do you spend any recreational time (*e.g.* hiking, jogging) along power line right-of-ways?

Rarely or never (0)   *Weekly (2)*   *Almost every day (4)* _____

12. Fluorescent lights give off higher fields than incandescent bulbs. Note how often you are in close proximity to fluorescent lights (1.5 m)?

Rarely or never (0)   *Weekly (2)*   *Almost every day (4)* _____

13. Do you place a motor-driven electric clock (*i.e.*, a plug-in clock with moving hands, as opposed to one with an LED/LCD display), a telephone answering machine or a portable fan within arm's reach of your bed?

No (0)   *Yes (3)*   _____

Add up the scores from all the questions to evaluate the category of your overall exposure.

Total number of points = ___22___

❖ If your score is below 16, then the total amount of fields encountered in your daily routine is below average.
❖ If your score is between 16 and 32, then the total amount of fields encountered in your daily routine is average.
❖ If your score is over 32, then the total amount of fields encountered in your daily routine is above average.

HISTORICAL SYNOPSIS

We have explored the many ways in which we encounter electromagnetic fields of various kinds in our daily lives. The focus of the next chapter is the scientific research on the interaction between weak electromagnetic fields and biological organisms. In order to provide a better sense of this issue, it is helpful to first provide a brief overview of the research and attendant controversy.

A discussion of the modern history of research into the biological effects of electromagnetic energy begins with the Soviet Union's efforts in the period after World War II. As the equipment to produce and measure microwaves, radio waves and other frequencies of electromagnetic waves improved, it became possible to carry out controlled scientific studies of cells, tissues and animals exposed to these waves. Western research focused on the idea of heating effects while Soviet scientists, who were interested in this too, looked into the possibility that levels below that required for heating could also have an effect.

In the 1950s, American scientist Herman P. Schwan developed an exposure limit for people exposed to microwaves in order to prevent heating effects. By 1965 this limit was adopted by the American National Standards Institute and authorities in other countries as an occupational exposure limit. There has always been some controversy surrounding this; for example, it has been pointed out that Schwan himself suggested that the limit was safe for probably no more than one hour.[7]

In 1968, the Soviet scientist A.S. Presman published a book, *Electromagnetism and Life,* in which he summarized several hundred research papers on electromagnetic field effects. Presman believed that the data of these numerous studies showed that electromagnetic energy could have effects even below heating levels. However, Presman's conclusion was rejected by most Western scientists.

By the 1970s only a limited amount of research had been carried out by Western scientists. In 1973, the U.S. military proposed building a communications network (codenamed "Sanguine") that would expose large numbers of people in Wisconsin to low-frequency electromagnetic fields. The scientists who reviewed the safety of this project raised several concerns about possible health effects, even on the basis of the limited data available at that time. They also suggested that if past studies showing bioeffects from low-frequency fields could be confirmed, perhaps the 60 Hz fields from such things as power lines should be investigated as potential public health factors.

Also during the 1970s, a series of public hearings on electric power transmission lines and the possibility of adverse health effects from them was undertaken in New York State. This led to the New York State Power Lines Project which began in 1981 and ended in 1987.

In the 1970s, few scientists took seriously this new type of research. It is fair to say that not many scientists even recognized that such research was being carried out.[8] Discussions of the possibility that exposure to low-intensity electromagnetic fields could have adverse health effects had captured little attention. Heating ability was considered the only valid criterion in the consideration of health effects from non-ionizing radiation.[9]

Project Sanguine and the New York State Public Service Commission hearings into a proposed new power line began to stir up some controversy, but it was not until 1979 that the issue of electromagnetic fields and health started to gain wider attention. Until that time Soviet studies and laboratory research on cells and animals exposed to electromagnetic fields formed the basis of the concerns of the few scientists who felt that electromagnetic fields may be environmental health factors.

Studies of humans are of course limited by ethical considerations. Evaluating risks due to various environmental factors such as water, air pollution or chemical contaminations is a part of a specialty called epidemiology. In epidemiological studies populations are examined in a way that will reveal risk factors associated with various life-threatening illnesses. In 1979, Dr. Nancy Wertheimer, an epidemiologist working in the area of childhood leukemia, published a study that was to fan the flames of controversy that were already smouldering. Armed with a list of childhood leukemia victims' addresses in Boulder, Colorado, Wertheimer visited these homes in the hope of discovering some common factor that might link the lives of these unfortunate children. In 1979, in association with physicist Ed Leeper, she published a study that suggested an increased risk of childhood leukemia for children whose homes were in close proximity to high-current electrical power lines. Considerable criticism was directed at this research but enough concern was generated for similar studies to be funded.

Within a few years the growing interest in this issue generated a series of epidemiological studies on electromagnetic fields and health. For example, a review of studies on electromagnetic fields and health in the workplace in 1991 listed some 63 studies carried out since 1980.[10] During the 1980s the public became increasingly aware of this issue. Power utilities sponsored their own studies. Given their role with respect to public electromagnetic field exposure, the validity of studies funded by utilities was questioned. The number of animal and cellular studies increased as more research money (and corresponding scientific interest) became available.

In 1989, the public was presented with a series of articles by *New Yorker* journalist Paul Brodeur. Brodeur, already well known for his involvement in bringing the controversy over asbestos to the public domain, galvanized concerns over environmental electromagnetic fields with his hard-hitting articles. Subsequent pieces in *Time* and *Business Week* also addressed electromagnetic fields, creating a higher profile for this issue. By 1990, after several decades of research which had received little attention and a lot of scepticism, the possibility that weak levels of non-ionizing fields may have a previously undiscovered relationship to human health was being taken more seriously.

The early 1990s have shown significant changes in attitudes towards this issue. The 1970s scepticism and lack of attention and the 1980s controversy and political posturing have given way to a "let's get down to research" attitude. The significant amount of research now accumulated has meant that an outright denial of biological effects from non-ionizing, non-thermal fields is no longer possible. A 1990 U.S. Environmental Protection Agency draft report even suggested that the evidence was strong enough to support a classification of "Class B carcinogen" for low-frequency magnetic fields. Although the final report removed this classification, that an authoritative organization could come to such a conclusion, even temporarily, is indicative of the changes that had taken place.

Other authoritative bodies now also conclude that non-thermal energy fields can have biological effects. The United States Office of Technology Assessment, for example, suggests in a 1989 report that non-thermal fields can interact with cells and tissues to produce changes. A 1991 British National Radiological Protection Board summary stated that not all electromagnetic field effects are attributable to heating. The American National Institute for Occupational Safety and Health (NIOSH) convened a meeting in January 1991, where researchers evaluated bioeffects from weak electromagnetic fields to establish what was known about electromagnetic fields in the workplace and to provide direction for future studies. This conference illustrated that although many outstanding questions remain, electromagnetic fields deserve attention as a possible workplace health concern.

Thus, weak electromagnetic energy fields are now seen as having the ability to produce changes in cells, tissues and animals. Two problems remain, however. First is the problem of how fields with so little energy can impact on a biological system. That is, what is (are) the mechanism(s) of action of weak electromagnetic energy fields? Until this problem is resolved, it is difficult to know which features of these fields are associated with biological changes, and scientists are reluctant to draw firm conclusions about weak fields as causal agents in epidemiological studies. Secondly, the important question remains as to whether significant risks to human health are associated with coming into contact with the fields from electric and electromagnetic technologies, both at home and in the workplace.

It is a difficult problem to elucidate the various risk factors of complex human illnesses such as cancer. While many epidemiological studies suggest a relationship between serious illnesses and electromagnetic fields, there are scientists who feel that something other than the energy fields may be the cause of the increases seen in these studies.[11] This is one of the many features of research that is part of the on-going scientific debate.

The present state of electromagnetic field research leaves unanswered questions. "More research!" is the call often sounded in this debate. One group of scientists feels that these fields should not, from a theoretical point of view, have biological activity and further research may show that something other than the fields are the cause of the positive results seen in some epidemiological studies. These scientists are increasingly in the minority. Another group of scientists feels that there is no doubt that weak electromagnetic energy fields can affect cells and tissues and that further research is required to more precisely define the risks to human health as required for public health policy. Since electromagnetic technologies have become virtual necessities, the problem remains to establish "acceptable" levels for the different types of electromagnetic energy fields, which is a process that is as much political as scientific. Let us now examine this process of research in more detail.

CHAPTER 2 NOTES

1. The smelting of aluminium requires large amounts of electricity, and aluminium smelters are typically located near hydroelectric projects. For example, in Kitimat, British Columbia, the Alcan corporation maintains its own hydro-generating facilities and sells power not required for aluminium smelting to BC Hydro, the public power utility. This electrical power will reach the plant as 60 Hz AC and is changed (rectified) to low voltage DC electricity. This electricity is then used to refine the aluminium. Currents of approximately 10,000 amperes can be found and magnetic fields of up to 800 gauss are produced.

2. Three examples of situations where household wiring can create above-average magnetic fields in your home are:

(i) If the wires are not laid out in pairs, and thus no magnetic field cancellation occurs.

ii) If some electrical wiring was carried out according to the local electrical code, but in a fashion that will not produce balanced (equal) current flow in the paired wiring. This kind of situation can be seen when there is more than one electrical panel in a home.

iii) Sometimes a situation can occur where the neutral current is unbalanced because some current returns to the utility pole through the grounding system.

3. The following figures are the power densities at various distances from a 50,000-watt AM radio station.

4.6 m	838 microwatt/cm^2
93.9 m	33 microwatt/cm^2
1000 m	1 microwatt/cm^2
1760 m	0.3 microwatt/cm^2

(From Tell, R. *et al.* (1979) "Electric and Magnetic Field Intensities and Associated Body Currents in Man in Close Proximity to a 50KW AM Standard Broadcast Station." Paper presented at Bioelectromagnetics Symposium, Seattle.)

4. Electric Power Research Institute (1990) "Electric and Magnetic Field Research." *EPRI Journal*, January/February.

5. Fisher, P.D. (1991) "Microwave Exposure Levels Encountered by Police Radar Operators. A Technical Report." East Lansing: Michigan State University.

6. Marino, A.A. (1988) "Environmental Electromagnetic Energy and

Public Health." In Marino, A.A., ed. *Modern Bioelectricity*. New York: Marcel Decker Inc., 965-1043.

7. Smith, C.W. and S. Best (1989) *Electromagnetic Man*. New York: St. Martin's Press.

8. Dr. Battocletti's 1976 book quoted in the introduction and Louise Young's 1974 discussion of power lines in the *Bulletin of Atomic Scientists* (December 1974, 34-38) represent early discussions of electromagnetic field and health concerns.

9. Even as early as 1969, in the introduction to Presman's book *Electromagnetism and Life*, the heat theory was referred to as a "Procrustean bed". This illustrates that some scientists, even at such an early stage, felt that the idea of heating could not explain all features of observed electromagnetic bioeffects.

10. National Institute for Occupational Safety and Health (1991) *Proceedings of the Scientific Workshop on Health Effects of Electric and Magnetic Fields on Workers* U.S. Department of Health and Human Services.

11. For example, living near a so-called high-current configuration power line has been associated with an increase in cases of childhood leukemia. However, it is possible that houses near such electrical configurations also tend to be closer to industrial districts with increased chemical contamination. This is one example of a hidden factor that may explain an observed increased leukemia risk, rather than actual electromagnetic fields. Hidden factors are often called confounders by epidemiologists. The whole picture of research has to be looked at, as even a very well carried out epidemiological study may have hidden factors that have been unaccounted for. Many confounders have been suggested for electromagnetic field-related epidemiology, but as of yet, none have been found to offer an alternative explanation other than that of implicating the electromagnetic fields themselves.

THREE

ELECTROMAGNETIC FIELDS AND BIOLOGY: THE UNFOLDING OF A NEW SCIENCE

Popular accounts of electromagnetic field research often describe results as "inconclusive" — especially, so it seems, when things might reflect badly on one of the many technologies that we so greatly enjoy. There is both truth and distortion in this description. Yes, there are many unanswered questions and much to learn about a new and challenging frontier of science. Yet at the same time, this obscures the fact that much has been learned in several decades of research. In this context, it is important to remember the fundamental uncertainties and ambiguities of all areas of science, and that all scientific theories are not ultimate truths; rather, they are temporary moments of consensus that are intimately linked to the culture at large of the time — the *Zeitgeist*. As Dr. Stephen Jay Gould, famous evolutionary biologist and historian of science, comments:

> *Science does, of course, seek truth; it even succeeds reasonably often, so far as we can tell. But science, like all of life, is filled*

with rich and complex ambiguity. The path to truth is rarely straight . . . Large numbers of little facts may eventually combine with other social and intellectual forces to topple a grand theory. The history of ideas is a play of complex human passions interacting with an external reality only slightly less intricate. We debase the richness of both nature and our own minds if we view the great pageant of our intellectual history as a compendium of new information leading from primal superstition to final exactitude.[1]

"Inconclusive" as electromagnetic bioeffects studies have been, they have observed effects not predicted by established theory. This poses a significant challenge to scientific orthodoxy, and this whole area of research has become highly controversial. It is fascinating to observe how each side of the debate is able to fit the results of each new study neatly (and often not so neatly) into their own framework. Gould, describing the intense debate between evolutionists and creationists of many shades in the 19th century, has pointed out with respect to a particular new discovery how "everyone made the best of it, incorporating favourable aspects of this new fact into his system and either ignoring or explaining away the difficulties."[1] The whole of the bioelectromagnetics research effort can be seen in this light: one group of scientists eagerly pushing forward with what they feel are exciting and important observations while another group denigrates their results as mistaken artifacts of the experimental process. And there are many shades of opinion lying somewhere in between.

The interpretive biases created by the uniquely coloured lenses of individual scientists are especially apparent in the case of the so-called literature review. Literature reviews are used to establish conclusions and form the basis for action. In a literature review those studies that have been carried out with the best preparation, planning and care are identified and from this selection, a picture of important developments and conclusions is drawn. This whole process leaves itself open to contradictory conclusions based on the same data. It is possible to pick and choose those studies that support preconceived ideas that a reviewer may have. Personal prejudices towards other researchers can enter into this process too.[2] When the conclusions of a scientific literature review have enormous implications for society, as is the case in electromagnetic field bioeffects research, it is not hard to imagine the "political science" that can go on behind the scenes.

It is difficult to fully present, in a single chapter, the scientific research that has been carried out in such a complex and multidisciplinary subject. This chapter emphasizes the dynamic process of research through a discussion of the three general categories of studies. The authors' bias enters through their choice of interesting examples of cellular, animal and epidemiological studies illustrating the research that has been carried out. The studies discussed in this chapter will not scratch the surface of the many scientific investigations carried out to date.[3] However, it is hoped that the reader will get some feeling for what the scientists, hidden away in laboratories all around the world, are working on.

The dynamic process of research can be understood as the interaction between three types of studies: *in vitro*, *in vivo*, and epidemiological. *In vitro* studies examine the effects of weak electromagnetic energy fields on simple cellular systems under rigorously controlled laboratory conditions. *In vivo* studies evaluate how weak electromagnetic energy fields interact with a more complex biological system — a whole animal — often using the basic principles of interaction learned from *in vitro* research. For example, if cells are found to be most sensitive to certain frequencies of weak electromagnetic fields, then these frequencies can be tested on animals. The animal models used in *in vivo* studies can help to provide information about how electromagnetic energy may affect our health, since studies on people are limited by ethical considerations.

Effective epidemiological studies can be carried out using the information gained from the two other types of scientific studies. Epidemiology studies large numbers of people to observe disease incidence and the various associated factors for these illnesses. The process of research can also move in the other direction: if epidemiologists are studying power frequency magnetic fields because public exposure to this frequency is common, laboratory studies of cells and animals can be most helpful if they also use fields of the same frequency. In fact, many cellular and animal studies have used the 50 Hz or 60 Hz power frequencies.

The development of new instrumentation also plays a role in this process. As an understanding of the interaction of weak fields with living things evolves, those parameters of the fields most important for determining the biological outcome can be uncovered. Instruments that can measure weak fields in the most biologically relevant way can be developed. For example, compact recording instruments have been designed so that they can be strapped to a worker's belt to measure exposure over a working day. Such instruments enable epidemiological studies to use measurements of exposure.[4]

As new insights are gained or as new questions emerge at one level of research, scientists respond by using this information or incorporating new questions into the design of future studies. Each new study adds another piece to the puzzle, and the whole process proceeds slowly — a single epidemiological study may take years from design to completion.

There is a real sense of excitement and drama surrounding this whole process. Those scientists studying cells are making observations that are not, according to conventional thinking, supposed to occur. Faced with limited funding and often a lack of support from their peers, these scientists are none the less pushing ahead to explore what they describe as one of the scientific frontiers of this century.

The search to observe previously unknown phenomena is also

joined with the job of explaining how these phenomena come about. New medical breakthroughs and a deeper understanding of the way in which living things work are goals of this flurry of activity. The excitement of this scientific frontier is perhaps overshadowed by the drama inherent in electromagnetic field epidemiology. As a result of the far-reaching consequences of the outcome of the epidemiological research, the results of each study become headline news and with public involvement and interest assured, the controversy of this new subject is heightened.

IN VITRO STUDIES

In vitro studies are carried out on cells or tissues in an artificial environment outside the living organism (*in vitro* means "in glass"). These cells can either be obtained from an animal of interest prior to experimentation, or can be special types of cells that are grown indefinitely in the laboratory. There are many advantages to studying cells or tissue outside the living organism. *In vitro* systems represent a simplification of more complex organisms. This allows the basic principles of interaction between weak electromagnetic energy fields and living things to be examined. Another very important advantage of an *in vitro* experiment is that a carefully designed laboratory environment can control the many experimental variables. That is, such things as temperature, humidity and electromagnetic field exposure can be accurately measured and maintained over the duration of an experiment. Without such precise control over all variables of an experiment, it is difficult to interpret the results. For example, changes in cell growth may have occurred from a temperature increase (if it was not held constant) and not from a magnetic field that was applied during a particular experiment.

In vitro experiments can be effectively repeated since essentially identical cells and conditions can be used. These experiments are much less costly than studies using animals or humans and are generally of much shorter duration. Theoretical models of the electromagnetic energy field interaction with cells are also easier.

Scientists hope that by studying these simpler cellular systems, the basic principles of the interaction between weak energy fields and living things can be understood. One major limitation of *in vitro* experimentation, however, is that the results and conclusions of studies carried out on cells in a test tube cannot easily be used to predict how humans or animals will respond to electromagnetic energy fields. This is due to the complexity of physiological systems composed of groups of cells which interact to make up a complete organism. *In vitro* experiments represent only one level of the overall effort to learn more about how weak electromagnetic energy fields can affect living things; other types of scientific research are still required to answer questions about human interactions with weak fields.

Examples of In Vitro Research

Many different features of cellular systems can be studied for changes in response to weak electromagnetic energy fields. The proliferation of cells *in vitro* can be affected by electromagnetic fields. The potential for clinical applications, including the use of low-frequency fields in the treatment of bone fractures that do not heal properly and tendinitis, has made this area of research particularly interesting. For example, Dr. Abraham Liboff found that by using low-frequency magnetic fields of the same strength that occur near fluorescent lights and electric motors, changes in the growth rate of human skin cells could be seen.[5] Increases of up to 100 per cent in DNA synthesis, which takes place as part of cell multiplication, were observed in these experiments.

Brain tissue has been studied *in vitro* to examine if the binding and release of calcium ions is affected by electromagnetic energy fields. This is a well-researched phenomenon and results have shown that brain tissues are indeed sensitive to very low intensities of electromagnetic energy fields. Calcium binding and release plays a role in neural processes,[6] so it is significant that electromagnetic energy fields can affect this physicochemical feature of tissue. Dr. W.R. Adey and Dr. Carl Blackman have studied the so-called calcium efflux phenomenon extensively; their work is described in more detail later in this section.

Cellular studies have demonstrated that weak electromagnetic energy fields can affect ribonucleic acid (RNA) transcription and protein synthesis. This is significant because these biomolecules are part of the basic chemical machinery of the cell. The work of Dr. Reba Goodman, who has examined *in vitro* changes of the cell's DNA and RNA due to weak electromagnetic energy field exposure, is discussed later in this section.

Dr. J.L. Phillips and his co-workers have provided yet another important study of electromagnetic energy field effects on cells.[7] Phillips and his team studied certain molecules called "receptors", found on the surface of the cell membrane where the cell interacts with other cells and the external environment. He found that when human colon cancer cells studied *in vitro* were exposed to 60 Hz electric and magnetic fields, there were changes in the expression of the transferrin receptor that was the focus of their investigation. The expression of this receptor is normally regulated as the number of cells in a colony increases, but Phillips found that field-exposed cells did not show such cell-density regulation even up to eight months after field exposure. He observed that 60 Hz electromagnetic fields could increase the formation of *in vitro* colonies of human colon cancer cells up to 24-fold. These results have led Phillips to postulate that low-frequency electromagnetic fields can interfere with the normal control mechanisms of cell growth.

Other researchers have examined whether weak electromagnetic energy fields can affect certain enzymes that are associated with cancer promotion (the second stage of the cancer process, following initiation). For example, C.V. Byus and his co-workers found a 500 per cent increase in the activity of one particular enzyme in human lymphoma cells studied *in vitro*.[8] This enzyme is important in regulating the growth of cells. Based on this and other results, Byus has suggested that 60 Hz electromagnetic fields may act as a tumour promoter.

Our immune system helps to defend against viruses and bacteria, and its role in preventing the excessive growth of cancerous cells continues to be investigated. The health of the immune system is intimately connected to the proper functioning of the whole body. It is of interest, then, to determine all the factors which might influence the immune system. Weak electromagnetic energy fields are now being studied in this context.

In vitro experiments with cellular components of the immune system have been carried out by D.B. Lyle and his co-workers.[9] These researchers found a 25 per cent reduction in the activity of the T-lymphocytes that were exposed to 60 Hz electric fields. T-lymphocytes are white blood cells that help to destroy antigens as part of an immune response. A reduced competency of the immune system due to electromagnetic fields may be related to the question of cancer.

Other researchers have also chosen T-lymphocytes to study immune system electromagnetic field effects.[10] Calcium plays an important role in acting as a signal between the exterior and the interior of the cell, and interference with the calcium signal has been shown to cause significant changes in cell behaviour. These researchers examined whether electromagnetic fields could influence the cell's immune response by producing changes in the calcium signal. They felt that if changes in calcium signalling could be observed, important features of the immune system may be influenced by electromagnetic fields.

The researchers' results were quite interesting. If the T-lymphocytes used in these studies did not have their calcium signalling stimulated, then the cells showed no response to weak fields. However, when the cells were activated by an immune-stimulating molecule, there was a response to electromagnetic fields. In one experiment, for example, the researchers observed a 2.4-fold increase in calcium transport after cells were immune-stimulated. If these same cells were exposed to 60 Hz fields, a 3.9-fold increase in calcium transport occurred after immune-stimulation of the cell. These results demonstrate once again that fields, theoretically too weak to be biologically important, can effect fundamental processes of living organisms. One of the scientists involved in this research, Dr. Jan Walleczek, suggests that weak electromagnetic fields may thus be able to influence human and animal immune responses. He mentions that six laboratories have in fact observed immune system changes in animals as a result of field exposure.

Again, it should be emphasised that these studies represent only a few selected examples of research. Another approach to the presentation of *in vitro* research is to feature a few of the prominent scientists in the field and the contributions they have made. Let us now discuss some of the research carried out by Dr. Reba Goodman, Dr. Carl Blackman and Dr. W.R. Adey.

Reba Goodman: Electromagnetic Field Effects on Protein Synthesis

Dr. Reba Goodman, a scientist at Columbia University, has published a number of papers with Dr. Ann Shirley-Henderson of the City University of New York, investigating the effects of low-frequency electromagnetic fields on cells.[11] These experiments have examined the workings of the basic biochemical machinery of the cell. The process of protein manufacture (protein synthesis) in a cell involves copying information from the DNA onto an RNA molecule. One type of RNA is called messenger RNA (mRNA) for its role in carrying information from the DNA to that region of the cell where protein synthesis takes place. Using different types of cells including a cultured line of human cells, Goodman and her colleagues found that exposure to low-frequency electromagnetic fields could increase the rate of messenger RNA transcription. These investigators also found changes in the patterns of protein synthesis, and observed new polypeptides (proteins) that were not detectable in unexposed cells. It is indeed interesting that inactive genes could be activated by electromagnetic fields; once again, fields that according to theory are too weak to influence biological systems, seem to be able to influence the most vital processes of living organisms.

All the messenger RNAs looked at in these studies showed similar patterns of response with respect to time and the strength of the applied field, and Goodman postulates that a general cellular mechanism is involved. Goodman's research helps confirm that low-intensity electromagnetic fields can indeed cause changes in cells, and demonstrates that changes in the most basic biochemical machinery can occur. It is this type of work that is forcing scientists to take a hard look at the past assumptions that weak fields were just that, too weak to be important. Clearly, the ability of weak fields to affect fundamental life processes means that these fields cannot be ignored *a priori* as environmental health factors.

Carl Blackman: Changes in Calcium Release from Brain Tissue

Another scientist who has studied the effects of electromagnetic fields on cellular systems and tissues *in vitro* is Dr. Carl Blackman, working at the Environmental Protection Agency's Health Effects Research Laboratory in North Carolina. Since 1979, Blackman and his colleagues have published a series of papers on the effects of low-intensity electromagnetic energy fields. During his decade and a half of research, Blackman has also written five scientific papers reviewing the biological effects of electromagnetic fields. In 1979, Blackman repeated experiments first carried out by Dr. W.R. Adey (discussed in the following section). Adey's experiments showed that the binding of calcium with brain tissue *in vitro* can be affected by low-frequency and amplitude-modulated[12] higher-frequency electromagnetic energy. In this case, the high-frequency radio waves were amplitude-modulated with low-frequency signals.

The changes in calcium binding to *in vitro* preparations of chicken brains, confirmed by Blackman in 1979, were apparently not due to heating of the tissue, as many scientists expected. Interestingly, the effects were related to the modulation frequency. Also, an enhanced outward flow (efflux) of calcium ions only occurred at certain intensities of the incoming modulated waves. This observation of frequency and intensity "windows" is one of the most interesting and puzzling features of biological responses to electromagnetic fields. (A "window" describes the fact that only specific intensity and frequency ranges were able to influence calcium binding.) Addressing the question of whether heating effects are involved in the calcium efflux phenomenon, Blackman concluded that "a solely thermal explanation appears extremely unlikely."[13] This is significant because, up until that time, this type of electromagnetic energy was thought to only influence biological systems by heating.

Blackman was interested to see if similar changes in calcium efflux would occur in brain tissue exposed to low-frequency electromagnetic fields without the high (radio) frequency component. In 1982, he published results showing that 16 Hz electromagnetic fields could change the calcium binding of brain tissue in the same way as was seen with higher frequency modulated radio waves. By 1985, this research was extended to show that a number of low frequencies can produce an efflux response. Blackman suggested that the response at 50 Hz (the European power frequency) seen in his experiments may explain effects reported by Soviet scientists.

In another 1985 paper, Blackman proposed an explanation for the fact that similar experiments carried out in different laboratories had produced conflicting results. The earth's magnetic field itself, Blackman suggested, may be an important hidden factor in the calcium efflux phenomenon.[14] If the earth's magnetic field plays a role, this could explain why different results were obtained in laboratories at different locations on the earth's surface, since the value of the geomagnetic field varies over the surface of the earth. This suggested a complex resonance phenomenon, whereby the earth's static field interacts with the applied low-frequency alternating field to produce the observed results. The mechanism of cyclotron resonance (discussed in the next chapter) describes such an interaction of the earth's magnetic field with an applied low-frequency field.

Another series of experiments carried out by Blackman's group deserves mention at this point. Chicken eggs were exposed during incubation to either 60 Hz or 50 Hz electric fields. After hatching, the brain tissues were observed for changes in the calcium efflux. Most interestingly, if eggs were exposed to 60 Hz electric fields during incubation, the brain tissue of the chickens hatched from the exposed egg showed an enhanced efflux at a frequency of 50 Hz but not at 60 Hz. However, after 50 Hz exposure of the eggs during incubation, the brain tissue of the hatched chicken did not show any changes in calcium efflux after either 50 Hz or 60 Hz exposure. As Blackman concludes, "these results demonstrate that exposure of a developing organism to ambient power-line-frequency electric fields at levels typically found inside buildings can alter the response of brain tissue to field-induced calcium-ion efflux."[15] He went on to add: "The physiological significance of this finding has yet to be established."

One important question for Blackman was whether these results carried out using tissues from chickens could be repeated in human cell culture systems. In 1989, Blackman working with Drs. S.K. Dutta and B. Ghosh from Howard University in Washington, D.C., showed that two different types of cells, both originating from the human central nervous system, were sensitive to radio-frequency waves. Thus, effects seen in chicken tissue could indeed be repeated in human cell systems.[16]

Later reports by Blackman extended studies on the role of the earth's magnetic field in the calcium efflux phenomenon,[17] and showed that calcium efflux could be very sensitive to temperature during exposure to weak energy fields.[18] Blackman continues to study the effects of electromagnetic fields on biological systems and to make a major contribution to this new field of endeavour.

W. Ross Adey: Bioelectromagnetics Pioneer

Dr. W. Ross Adey is another important researcher investigating the effects of weak electromagnetic energy fields on biological systems. He is also one of the most outspoken defenders of the idea that sub-thermal levels of electromagnetic energy can affect cells, tissues and organisms. Adey feels that the study of the role of electromagnetic energy in living things is "one of the most significant new scientific frontiers of this century, pointing the way to an understanding of the essence of living matter in physical mechanisms at the atomic level."[19]

Adey deserves mention not only for the experimental studies he has been involved in for over two decades, but for his synthesis of ideas from a wide range of scientific disciplines. He has used frontier developments in areas such as condensed matter physics, the pathology of cancer, brain physiology, and cell membrane biophysics to push forward the understanding of the basic processes of living things and to overcome the limitations of current theoretical concepts.

Adey has been frustrated by the political dimensions surrounding bioelectromagnetics research and points out that the potential for new developments in biology has been hindered by the reluctance of many scientists to give up their attachment to inappropriate theoretical approaches. In a 1991 article in *Environmental Health Perspectives*, referring to the electromagnetic fields and health controversy, Adey states, "much has been accomplished in the past decade in establishing a firm base of new knowledge, despite a grave and growing lack of research funds and also entrenched and often self-serving attitudes among influential groups who have denied the possibility of adverse effects, based simply on their *a priori* positions."[20]

Adey points out that engineers have only been concerned with the heating effects, so they assume that any level of exposure not capable of heating should be safe. Physiologists have denied the potential importance of weak electromagnetic fields since traditional models of cell membrane physiology do not predict any effects from these fields. Adey also criticizes physicists who maintain that the low energy of the fields studied should not affect biological matter because of the problem of thermal noise (discussed in the next chapter). He suggests that such objectors should become better informed of the many new discoveries in physics that could provide a physical understanding of electromagnetic field effects on biological systems. Let us explore some of Adey's research and ideas.[21]

In the late 1970s Adey, working with Dr. Susan Bawin, was the first to demonstrate that weak electromagnetic fields could change the binding of calcium to brain tissue *in vitro*.[22] The experiments of Adey and Bawin demonstrated that electromagnetic fields, at extra-low and amplitude-modulated radio frequencies, were able to produce changes in calcium binding. Certain frequencies and amplitudes of the electromagnetic fields were more effective than others. Adey and Bawin explained the significance of these results in terms of an interaction of the applied fields with binding sites on the surface of the cell membrane. The important role of the cell membrane in communication between the outside and the inside of the cell, and the key role calcium plays in many physiological processes, suggests that this observation may provide an insight into the inner workings of cell function.

With a broad perspective, Adey has written many articles reviewing the current knowledge of the interaction between weak electromagnetic fields and living things. He has been outspoken about the potential significance of this new field of endeavour. For example, in a 1981 review, Adey suggests that the use of weak fields to probe biological units at the molecular level will assist in the study of normal and abnormal growth processes, the function of the immune system, and cellular communications.[23] Adey emphasizes that the kinds of processes that electromagnetic fields seem to interact with are "cooperative" in nature and cannot be understood in terms of the models presently used to describe biological systems. This cooperative nature is seen in the low levels of energy that are required to activate a response and the fact that only certain frequencies and intensities are effective at doing so.

In response to the success of using weak energy fields to stimulate the repair of bone fractures that weren't healing normally, Adey and his co-workers published a paper in 1982 showing the results of experiments on the bone cells of mice *in vitro*.[24] They observed changes in a number of cellular biochemical parameters and concluded that the observed effects may have been due to interference with the interaction of hormones at the surface of the cell membrane. In other 1982 publications, Adey described results showing that the calcium efflux phenomenon could also be observed in cats which were immobilized under local anaesthesia. He also described a theoretical model, using nonlinear wave mechanics, that could be applied to membrane processes whereby electromagnetic fields could have effects on the membrane even at low energies.

In 1987, Adey reviewed the evidence that weak electromagnetic fields play a role in cancer promotion.[25] He concluded that the cell membrane is the major site of interaction between the fields and living tissue, and that electromagnetic energy could influence the signals sent from cell surface receptors to the cell interior. Cell surface receptors respond to hormones, antibodies, neurotransmitters and also chemical cancer promoters. Thus, Adey postulated, cancer promotion may be made possible by the synergistic action of electromagnetic energy fields and cancer-promoting agents. This could occur by interference with the signals sent from the cell surface to the nucleus and organelles present inside the cell.

Adey suggests a three-stage model for the biological effects of electromagnetic fields at intensities below that required for heating. This model involves the process of signals being sent from the exterior to the interior of a cell. First, at the surface of the membrane there exist highly charged protein molecules which are sensitive to electromagnetic energy fields and to the binding of hormones and neurotransmitters at cell surface receptors. Secondly, these protein molecules have sections that traverse the membrane and penetrate into the cell interior, thereby providing a means for the surface influence of electromagnetic fields to be transmitted to the cell interior. Finally, the signals can influence enzyme systems inside the cell or travel to the cell nucleus, thereby having an effect on cell function. Adey concludes this paper with the suggestion that "it is at the atomic level that physical, rather than chemical events now appear to shape the flow of signals and the transmission of energy on biomolecular systems. Recent observations have opened doors to new concepts of communication between cells as they whisper together across barriers of cell membranes."[26]

Working with Dr. Larry Anderson and other researchers, Adey investigated the influence of electromagnetic fields on the daily rhythms of brain neurotransmitters and enzymes in rats.[27] Also in the late 1980s, Adey worked with other researchers investigating the influence of electromagnetic energy on important cellular enzymes.[28] For example, the enzyme ornithine decarboxylase has been shown to have an enhanced level of activity in growing cells and tissues and during the process of tumour promotion. Their studies demonstrated that the activity of this enzyme could be activated by exposure to 60 Hz fields. Adey's research in the 1990s has included involvement in studies dealing with the prenatal exposure of rats to low-frequency fields, and using electromagnetic fields as a tool to investigate animal models of epilepsy. Adey continues to be actively involved in this new scientific frontier.

IN VIVO STUDIES

While research using cells has many advantages, it is important to study the effects of electromagnetic energy fields on animals or people. This is because it is too difficult to predict on the basis of studies of isolated cells how animals or people will be affected.

Ethical considerations limit the use of people in scientific research to mainly epidemiological surveys. Animals thus provide the most direct models for studies of more complex systems.[29] Although extrapolation of the results of animal studies to human exposure conditions is often tenuous, experiments on animals are important in extending cellular studies and in providing a firm basis for understanding human effects. A variety of animals have served as subjects for research, ranging from commonly used rats and mice to dogs, pigs, cats and monkeys.

Different features of animal anatomy, physiology and behaviour have been examined for responses to fields. Animal behaviour is highly sensitive to environmental influences, and a number of researchers have studied behavioral changes in response to electromagnetic field exposure.

Scientists have studied the effects of electromagnetic fields on neurotransmitters, important chemical components of the nervous system. They have often chosen neurotransmitters that are associated with the so-called stress response. Also of interest is the effect of weak electromagnetic fields on reproduction and development. In early stages of development, animals are considered to be most sensitive to possible environmental stresses such as chemicals or electromagnetic fields. As will be discussed, studies on the incidence of malformation in chicken eggs provide an example of this category of inquiry.

Bone growth and repair has been studied. This is of interest since the use of pulsed magnetic fields to stimulate the regrowth of non-unionized bone fractures is now a clinical technique used by medical practitioners. Interestingly, pulsed magnetic fields appear to improve the rate of healing, while sinusoidal electric fields in some experiments show a negative effect on bone repair. ("Pulsed" and "sinusoidal" describe the way in which the fields change in time.) Studies on both the cardiovascular system and immune system of animals have been carried out. One important area of research is the study of electromagnetic fields on biological rhythms. A few studies have looked at the questions of cancer and genetic mutations in animals. This is of particular interest as the number of epidemiological studies suggesting an association between cancer and electromagnetic fields are increasing. At a 1991 conference sponsored by the National Institute of Occupational Safety and Health (NIOSH), it was recommended that researchers "diligently pursue" the question of a role for electromagnetic fields in the development of cancer.[30]

Early Examples of Animal Research

The earliest animal experiments, for the most part, focused on the heating effects of radio and microwave fields and the effects of strong low-frequency electric fields.[31] For example, a study published in 1980 by a research group including Dr. Robert Becker and Dr. Andrew Marino at the Veterans Administration Medical Centre in Syracuse, New York, reported a study on biological changes in successive generations of mice exposed to strong 60 Hz electric fields. This report was motivated by the possible health consequences of public exposures to power-frequency (60 Hz) electric fields. Becker and Marino noted that until the mechanisms of interaction between electromagnetic fields and living systems were better understood, animal studies will be required to help develop human exposure standards. They concluded that exposures to strong electric fields caused an increased mortality rate in each generation, and by the third generation, increased body weights were observed in the exposed mice. The authors discussed their findings in terms of a stress model, considering the applied electric field as a stressor.[32]

Another example of an early animal study was reported in

1976 in the journal *Nature* by scientists at the University of California at Los Angeles.[33] Changes in monkey behaviour were observed as a result of exposure to weak electric fields. This experiment was unusual, since most researchers were more interested in effects of stronger electric fields. In the UCLA experiments, monkeys were trained to press a lever on a schedule, and changes in the time between lever presses were measured. The authors found that the time between lever presses could be affected by exposing the monkeys to weak low-frequency electric fields. In their report, the authors drew attention to the fact that other examples of biological effects from weak electromagnetic energy fields existed at that time. These included the observation of magnetic field effects on homing pigeons, the use of electric fields by fish to detect their prey, and the influence of 10 Hz electric fields on human circadian rhythms.

Before 1980 few researchers were interested in the effects of low-frequency magnetic fields on animals. One exception was a 1975 report by Japanese researchers studying the effects of 50 Hz fields on experimentally induced arthritis in rats.[34] Improvement of the arthritis in the rats' forepaws was observed in this study after exposure to 50 Hz magnetic fields. In their paper, these scientists noted that the treatment of rheumatic and inflammatory disorders with magnetic fields is common in Japan.

Electromagnetic Fields and Biological Rhythms in Animals

All organisms demonstrate rhythmic patterns in biological processes. Especially important are the daily (circadian) changes. These rhythms, connected to the basic processes of a living organism, respond to environmental signals. There are several features of circadian rhythms that can be altered.[35] Alterations in our rhythms are associated with biochemical and physiological changes and can be related to changes in our health. For example, changes in daily cycles have been correlated with psychological depression and weakening of the immune system.

Because of the importance of circadian rhythms and their sensitivity to environmental influences, a number of scientists have studied the effects that electromagnetic fields have on these cycles. A major focus of these studies has been biochemical changes in the pineal gland, which plays a role in secreting a number of physiologically important biochemicals including the hormone melatonin, thereby helping to control the circadian rhythms. Studies have included observations of daily changes in an organism's activity, energy consumption and body temperature.

For example, Drs. F.M. Sulzman and D.E. Murrish studied the relationship between power line fields and behavioural changes associated with circadian rhythms in monkeys.[36] These researchers exposed monkeys to electric and magnetic fields and observed their behaviour for both acute and chronic changes. The monkey's circadian cycles were found to be affected by field exposure.

A number of scientists have measured changes in the daily rhythms of the secretions of the pineal gland after animals were exposed to electromagnetic fields. For example, the pineal gland secretes melatonin, a hormone that plays a key role in regulating the activity of the brain. Wilson and his colleagues observed a marked decrease in the normal nighttime rise of melatonin and other pineal secretions in rats after they were exposed to electric fields. This decrease occurred after several weeks of chronic exposure.[37] Other scientists have shown that magnetic fields and even an alteration in the normal geomagnetic field can affect circadian features of pineal secretions.[38] In the words of one bioelectromagnetics reviewer:

Although firm conclusions cannot yet be made regarding potential health impacts from [extra low frequency] effects on circadian biological rhythms, it is apparent that [electromagnetic] fields can alter the circadian timing mechanisms in mammals.[30]

The panel of scientists assembled for a 1991 NIOSH conference felt that one of the most interesting *in vivo* findings was the ability of low-frequency electromagnetic fields to inhibit the nighttime synthesis of the hormone melatonin in the rodent pineal gland. In a summary of research recommendations, these scientists suggested that inhibition of melatonin synthesis may form a basis for a plausible mechanism associating cancer with electromagnetic fields. Electromagnetic field-induced hormonal changes may also provide a link to effects on reproduction and development.[30]

Developmental Studies

One area of focus for bioelectromagnetics scientists has been the effects of electromagnetic fields on reproductive and developmental features of animals. The greater sensitivity of animals to environmental stresses in the early stages of life suggests that electromagnetic field effects may be more readily observed in developing animals. Another reason for interest in this area is the concern about effects of electromagnetic fields on pregnant women from field sources such as electric blankets and computer video display terminals (VDTs). As a result, studies of developing mammals and birds have been carried out in a number of laboratories.

One example of this type of study was carried out in 1990 by Kurt Salzinger and his co-workers at the Polytechnic University in Brooklyn.[39] Their study looked at rats that were exposed to electric and magnetic fields during gestation and the first eight days after birth. Later, as adults, these same rats were tested for their response to behavioural conditioning. The conditioning involved the rewarding of food for pressing a lever. Interestingly, the rats exposed in their early stages of development "responded at significantly lower rates" than identical rats that were not exposed.[39]

In a 1982 paper, the Spanish scientist José M.R. Delgado, working with a group of researchers in Madrid, published the results of experiments that were to capture interest worldwide.[40] Using the development of fertilized chicken eggs as a model to study the effects of magnetic fields, Delgado's team observed changes in the exposed chicken eggs. Over the course of the experiments, the effects of pulsed magnetic fields of different frequencies and intensities were tested on the eggs. The results showed that some frequencies and intensities were more likely to produce abnormalities than others. This was the same type of "window" effect that had been previously observed in Ross Adey's calcium binding studies of chicken brain tissue. In the group of eggs not exposed to fields, over 80 per cent showed normal development, but almost 80 per cent of the exposed eggs showed detectable abnormalities. The scientists described the effects of magnetic field exposure as an inhibition of embryogenesis. They concluded that low-intensity (low-frequency) magnetic fields may be a useful tool to study embryogenetic mechanisms.

An important part of the scientific process is the ability of other laboratories to corroborate the conclusions of important experiments. The Delgado study was repeated in six laboratories around the world — in Canada, the United States, Sweden and Spain. In five of the six laboratories, exposed eggs showed a higher percentage of abnormalities than similar non-exposed eggs. Combining the results of all laboratories, eggs exposed to pulsed low-frequency magnetic fields showed a 25 per cent incidence of abnormalities while 19 per cent of non-exposed eggs demonstrated abnormalities.[41]

Animal Experiments Using Radio/Microwaves

While lower-frequency electric and magnetic fields have been used in studies on animals, there has also been interest in whether higher-frequency non-ionizing fields can affect animals. Earlier animal studies have monitored the heating effects from radio and microwave exposure. The heating effects of higher intensities of radio and microwaves are used as a basis for protection guidelines. The controversial aspect, however, is whether intensities of radio and microwaves below that required for heating can also cause biological effects.

Several experiments using modulated radio frequency waves were mentioned in the *in vitro* section. In a 1989 article entitled "Biological Effects of Radiofrequency Radiation: An Overview," Dr. Stephen F. Cleary provides eleven different examples of effects of radio frequency fields on cellular systems at levels below that required for heating.[42] In his review, Cleary states:

> *Review of the bioeffects literature, especially the results of in vitro cellular studies provides convincing evidence that [radio frequency] radiation, and other types of electric or magnetic fields, can alter living systems via direct nonthermal mechanisms, as well as via heating.*[42]

The observation that higher-frequency fields can affect cellular systems suggests the importance of using animal studies, since these cellular effects cannot directly be used to understand how animals or humans will be affected by radio and microwaves. Of particular interest has been the possibility of a relationship between radio and microwave fields and the process of cancer development. As an example, an Environmental Protection Agency (EPA) review noted that experiments by the Polish scientist Stanislaw Szmigielski demonstrated that exposing mice to microwaves may stimulate the growth of tumours and act as a tumour promoter.[43] It is not clear whether tissue heating played a role in these observations — remember that radio and microwaves are capable of heating tissues at higher intensities.

In his experiments, Szmigielski exposed mice continuously to microwaves for several months and found an acceleration of the appearance and growth of chemically induced cancers. Szmigielski suggests that his limited data demonstrating a cancer-promoting action may be due to either a direct effect at the cellular level or an indirect action of immune system suppression.[42]

Another study discussed in the EPA review involved the long-term exposure of rats to (pulsed) microwave fields. The EPA suggested that this study, carried out by Dr. Bill Guy at the University of Washington, may provide evidence that such fields could cause cancers in a non-specific way. Different parts of the rat's body showed statistically significant increases in carcinomas even without appreciable tissue heating. This study was done using a microwave intensity equal to the maximum allowable level for continuous human exposure set by the American National Standards Institute (ANSI).[42,43]

EPIDEMIOLOGICAL STUDIES

Cellular and animal studies represent just one facet of electromagnetic field research. While these studies help to elucidate basic principles of interaction between electromagnetic fields and living things, the question of human health effects requires a more direct evaluation. Actual experiments on humans are, of course, restricted, so it is epidemiological investigations that provide information on the relationship between electromagnetic fields and human health.

Epidemiology is a branch of medical science which evaluates the many factors that are associated with human disease. Epidemiological studies are essentially statistical in nature, usually examining large numbers of people, and the associations between various measures of human health and the factors that may play a role in the disease process. Examples of factors include such things as exposure to environmental chemical contaminants, smoking, and aspects of diet.

An epidemiological study may generate a hypothesis by, for example, searching through registries of morbidity and finding associations between certain occupations and specific illnesses. Hypothesis generation is one kind of epidemiological study. Another type of epidemiological investigation may involve testing a hypothesis. For example, if an association between electromagnetic field exposure and childhood leukemia is postulated, this could be studied by comparing the electromagnetic field exposure of children with leukemia to that of a group of children without leukemia. This so-called case-control study is a more powerful statistical method of evaluating the importance of risk factors for human diseases.

These first two types of studies are both retrospective studies in the sense that information from the past must be used as part of the evaluation. For example, in a case-control study examining childhood leukemia and electromagnetic field exposure, a child's electromagnetic field exposure in the past has to be ascertained. This exposure history may be complicated by such things as changing residences or lifestyle patterns.

So-called prospective studies are an attempt to overcome this difficulty. In a prospective study, a group of people is followed over a period of time, and both the incidence of specific illnesses and information on the hypothesized risk factor can be obtained during the study. Such a study can more accurately obtain information on the risk factor(s) of interest. However, a large group of people must be followed for a significant length of time, especially when dealing with rare illnesses. One type of prospective study is a cohort study, in which a defined group of people is the focus of investigation.

Such epidemiological investigations hope to determine the relative risk associated with a specific disease factor. Depending on the design of the study, there are a number of statistical indicators that may be evaluated.[44] Epidemiological studies may use the fact that certain groups of people are exposed to electromagnetic fields to an extent greater than is normal (all members of the public are exposed to electromagnetic fields to some extent). The degree of certain illnesses in these exposed groups can be compared to similar groups of unexposed people, or to the overall level of these illnesses in the general population. In the example of a case-control study, already discussed, a group of people with a certain disease can have their electromagnetic field exposure contrasted to a group without the disease.

It should be stressed that while epidemiological investigations can show associations between a factor and a disease, an association does not prove a causal link. Epidemiologists are always careful to point to the difference between association and causation. In order to establish causation after a demonstration of association, scientists evaluate a number of features of the proposed relationship. These include: the strength of the observed relationship; the consistency of the observations (repetition in different studies); the plausibility of causality (which is influenced by the theoretical expectations prevalent at the time of the study); analogy (are there other similar examples?); the probability that the outcome could have occurred by chance; and the dose-response (does more exposure to the factor result in higher occurrence of the disease?).

Many of these are subjective and open for interpretation; there is no clear point in epidemiological research where causality is objectively demonstrated. Rather, there is a process of debate, research to eliminate viable alternative hypotheses, and related cellular and animal research to confirm the plausibility of causality. This helps to explain why many epidemiological investigations have shown associations between electromagnetic fields and human ill-health, yet there is so much debate.

Diseases like cancer are complex, often having long periods of development following induction, and with many etiological factors. This adds to the difficulty in carrying out epidemiological research. Further, the basic parameters of electromagnetic fields (intensity, frequency, etc.) that should be measured for use in epidemiological surveys are far from being understood. Cellular and developmental studies indicate that electromagnetic field interactions may not follow a usual dose-response relationship (*i.e.*, twice the amount of exposure may not yield twice the effect). Whether unusual features of interaction, such as amplitude and frequency windows,[45] have implications for human exposures is now the focus of research. This incomplete understanding of the biological basis of electromagnetic field effects helps to explain the highly controversial nature of such studies. Also, undoubtedly, something with as far-reaching consequences as an association of low-intensity electromagnetic field exposure with human illness creates a scientific scrutiny and burden of proof greatly exceeding that normally seen.

This process of inquiry proceeds slowly, especially given the limited funding available for electromagnetic field research. These difficulties are not presented to suggest that the whole field of inquiry is somehow vague and uncertain. Rather, they help us understand the true picture of the research effort. It should be emphasized that all new areas of study in science are also characterized by a host of difficulties not unlike the present case. The example of the study of smoking as a health factor is a case in point that is discussed further at the end of this chapter. Thus, uncertainties are to be expected and are what drive the search to learn more. At the same time electromagnetic field research is becoming more important; scientific and public opinion has changed drastically in the past decade; and more and more epidemiological studies are implicating electromagnetic fields as risk factors for human illnesses.

A lot of epidemiological work has focused on individuals who work in places that can be described as electrical environments. Occupational electromagnetic field epidemiology represents the most examined area, and many studies of this kind are presently under way. Studies of the association of childhood leukemia and electromagnetic field exposure from power lines have caught the most public attention. Other studies have investigated birth outcome among electrically heated waterbed and electric blanket users, as well as in the families of workers whose job exposes them to electromagnetic fields. For example, the incidence of cancers in the central nervous system (such as brain cancer) has been examined in children whose fathers were occupationally exposed to electromagnetic fields before the child's birth. Other health parameters such as suicide and depression have been studied for a link with electromagnetic fields. And interestingly, though not epidemiological research, some scientists and medical practitioners suggest that there are individuals who are allergic to electromagnetic fields. This allergic reaction has been called the "electromagnetic hypersensitivity syndrome."[46] Let us present examples of these studies and discuss the general conclusions of the results to date.[47]

Occupational Electromagnetic Field Epidemiology

The epidemiological association of cancer with electromagnetic fields by Dr. Nancy Wertheimer in 1979 stimulated an interest in occupational electromagnetic fields as a possible risk factor for human diseases. Many types of cancers are now being studied in occupational electromagnetic field epidemiology. Different kinds of leukemia, brain cancer, skin cancer and male breast cancer are all outcomes that have been examined for an association with electromagnetic field exposure on the job. These studies for the most part did not use actual measurements of electromagnetic fields but instead used surrogates, for example job descriptions, to provide an indication of exposure.

A number of studies have examined the relationship between low-frequency fields and leukemia. The majority of the twelve hypothesis-generating studies carried out between 1982 and 1988 suggested a positive association (see Figure 3). However, these studies had many weaknesses, and they needed to be combined with more powerful examinations of the electromagnetic field/cancer relationship. In fact, case-control studies of leukemia among workers have been carried out. The results of these more powerful studies lend support to an association between leukemia and electrical occupations. However, the major limitation is that actual measurements of electromagnetic fields were not used. A similar conclusion has been made for case-control studies of brain cancer.[48]

Cohort studies of electrical workers also have shown positive associations between electrical occupations and cancer, especially skin melanoma. Dr. Gilles Theriault, an authority on electromagnetic field epidemiology, points out that as the groups of workers exposed to electromagnetic fields have been categorized with greater precision, stronger associations of electromagnetic fields with leukemia and brain cancer have been observed.[48] One

area of concern noted by epidemiologists is a possible association of parental occupational electromagnetic field exposures

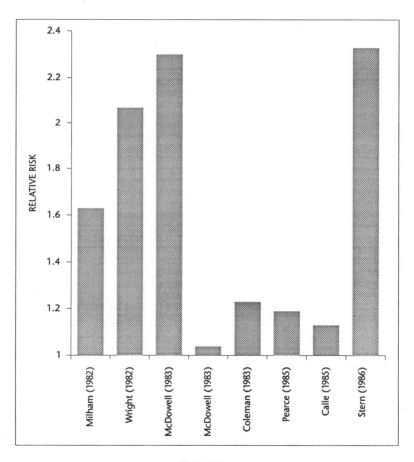

FIGURE 3

Between 1982 and 1986, eight studies reported on the risk of leukaemia
faced by men working in various "electrical occupations." Coleman and
Beral combined the results of these studies and calculated a relative risk
of about 1.5. Adapted from: Coleman, M. and V. Beral, *Int. J. Epid.* 1988.
Vol. 17:1 - 13.

and brain cancer in their offspring. This is something that will undoubtedly get more attention in future investigations.

A number of studies have reported associations with male breast cancer, a very rare illness.[48,49] Some scientists feel that this is significant because breast cancer has a hormonal connection and electromagnetic fields have been shown to affect the hormonal system, especially the important hormone melatonin.

This connection of electromagnetic fields to hormonal effects also suggests that electromagnetic fields may be a factor in psychological disorders such as depression and suicide. In a 1988 paper, Dr. Bary Wilson discussed the connection of low-frequency fields to depression.[50] He noted that several studies have correlated the incidence of depression-related suicide with electromagnetic fields. Wilson described the effects that low-frequency fields could have on circadian rhythms of melatonin concentration in rats. He suggested a link to depressive disorders in human beings by noting that alterations in the circadian rhythms of melatonin secretion are in fact associated with these types of psychiatric illnesses. According to Wilson, if chronic exposure to fields causes problems in the human pineal gland as it does in rats, these biochemical changes may help to bring on depression or worsen already existing conditions.

What conclusions can be drawn from epidemiology about the relationship between cancer and occupational electromagnetic field exposure? This question was addressed by Gilles Theriault at the Scientific Workshop on the Health Effects of Electric and Magnetic Fields on Workers in 1991:

> *Almost all "electrical occupations" have shown excesses of one cancer or another but no consistent observation has allowed firm conclusions. The size of the excess risk noted so far may seem small but it is to be regarded seriously in view of the poor estimates of exposure used. The real agent responsible for the excesses of cancer observed in "electrical occupations" may be something other than [electromagnetic fields] (referred to as confounders by many authors), such as chemical exposures, but*

this has yet to be demonstrated . . . one cannot help from recognizing that the evidence points toward the existence of one carcinogenic factor in "electrical occupations and/or environment."[48]

A similar conclusion was drawn by the New York State Power Lines Project scientific advisory panel's final report in July of 1987:

Despite the obvious limitations of these studies and the erratic findings, it is difficult to avoid the conclusion that there is a certain consistency between the results. It seems more likely that these occupations are at an increased risk of leukemia than that a random phenomenon is observed or that some sort of bias is operating. If these "electrical" occupations are in fact at increased risk, whether or not the explanation is known, then it seems warranted to include long-term exposure to magnetic fields on the candidate list.[51]

Studies on Reproductive Effects

Interest in the interaction between electromagnetic fields and human reproduction and development has led to several studies. One controversial area has been the relationship between computer video displays and the risk of miscarriage. Let us examine two examples of this research.

Since her ground-breaking epidemiological survey of childhood leukemia in 1979, Dr. Nancy Wertheimer has continued to study the electromagnetic field and health question. In a paper published in 1986 with physicist Ed Leeper in the journal *Bioelectromagnetics*, Wertheimer addressed the question of reproductive effects from the use of electric bedding devices.[52] The paper, "Possible Effects of Electric Blankets and Heated Waterbeds on Fetal Development," opens with the observation that since earlier studies indicate that heat or electromagnetic fields produced by waterbeds and electric blankets might affect the fetus, it is important to study pregnancy outcomes in users of these devices.

The study looked at the length of the gestation period, birth weight, and (favourable/unfavourable) outcome of pregnancy. The data were analyzed on a month-by-month basis because in Denver, Colorado, where the study was carried out, electric blankets and waterbed heaters are used extensively in the cold winter months and not at all in the summer months, while both spring and fall use lies somewhere in between.

Wertheimer's study found that users of electric blankets and heated waterbeds showed a distinct seasonal variation in gestation time and the number of miscarriages, whereas women who did not use these devices showed no variation. Interestingly, miscarriages among users of electrical bedding devices were highest from September through January, and not over the period of heaviest use during the coldest months of the year, as might be first expected. Wertheimer explains that during September to January, the number of cold nights is increasing so a fetus would be exposed to the increasing use of bedding heating systems. Thus, she states that the seasonal variation of reproductive indicators is strongly associated with the *changes* in temperature seen from month to month and not the temperature itself. Hence, it appears that these reproductive indicators are most sensitive to *changes* in exposure to heat or electromagnetic fields and not to the absolute level of the heat or fields themselves.

Wertheimer noted that earlier studies showed that chicken embryos exposed to electromagnetic fields at high temperatures developed abnormalities, while those exposed to the same fields at low temperatures did not. This was of interest because electrical bedding devices produce both heat and electromagnetic fields.

In addressing a possible mechanism for this observation, Wertheimer noted that the embryos generate their own internal electrical currents that may play a role in embryogenesis, and proposed that external electromagnetic fields create electrical currents that may interfere with the embryo's endogenous currents. It is also possible that the reproductive effects seen were entirely due to the influence of heat on fetal development. However, as Wertheimer and Leeper conclude:

Whatever mechanism, it seems important to study the possibility of adverse effects from electric bed heaters further, since their use seems to be increasing as the cost of home heating rises. Possibly such increased use contributes to the unexplained increase in childhood disability reported to have occurred since 1960, especially among the nonpoor.[52]

The possibility of a link between electromagnetic fields from computer displays (VDTs) and risk of miscarriage has been a controversial topic for some time. Psychological stresses and ergonomic considerations have also been proposed as possible factors associated with pregnancy outcome among computer users. Many of the studies to date have evaluated the amount of time spent working at a computer VDT, and have found no association.

A recent study carried out in Finland improved on the design of previous research by measuring the low-frequency magnetic fields of the women's computer VDTs. They included this information along with job stress and ergonomic factors in their analysis. Dr. Marja-Liisa Lindbohm's paper, published in a 1992 issue of the *American Journal of Epidemiology* under the title "Magnetic Fields of Video Display Terminals and Spontaneous Abortion,"[53] reported that no increased risk of miscarriage occurred when comparing women who frequently used VDTs (20 hours per week or more) to those with infrequent use (10 hours per week or less). However, when women using VDTs emitting high levels of low-frequency magnetic fields were compared to those using units producing much lower levels of these fields, miscarriages were more than three times as likely to occur in the high-field group. Lindbohm ends her paper by calling for more research on the effects of low-frequency magnetic fields on pregnancy outcome, and that this research should use measurements of the fields in the actual workplace (Lindbohm's study recorded magnetic field levels in a laboratory for the different models of VDTs). Lindbohm also noted that female employees in industrial and other electrical environments should be studied.

Childhood Leukemia and Power Lines

It was Dr. Nancy Wertheimer's 1979 study of childhood leukemia and power line magnetic fields that helped alert the public — and many scientists — to the possibility that our use of electricity poses a health hazard.

The Wertheimer study used a system, called wire coding, of classifying electrical utility lines near a child's residence as a means of estimating the magnetic field exposures. With the wire coding approach, magnetic fields are not actually measured, but estimated on the basis of an examination of possible magnetic field sources. Because magnetic fields are related to electrical current, Wertheimer's team could look at the wires around a child's home and make a judgment as to the amount of current they carry; then use this judgment of current to estimate the releative strength of the magnetic fields that would be created. Her study found a two-fold increase in leukemia risk for children whose homes were located near so-called high-current configuration power lines.[54]

The study's methods have been criticized on at least two grounds. Firstly, magnetic fields from other sources such as appliances and unbalanced ground return currents are not considered in the wire coding approach — only power lines. Secondly, there has been some question as to whether wire coding has a direct relationship to actual measurements of magnetic fields.

As part of the New York State Power Lines Project (NYSPLP), epidemiologist Dr. David Savitz repeated and improved upon the design of the Wertheimer study. For example, both direct measurements of electromagnetic fields and Wertheimer's wire coding system of classifying utility lines were used in the Savitz study published in 1986. In order to ensure the effectiveness of the study, Savitz gave the participants in the study a question-naire to help account for other factors (called confounders[55]) that might influence the results, such as X-ray exposure or smok-ing. With these improvements, the Savitz study again saw an in-creased risk of leukemia for children living in close proximity to high-current configuration power lines as compared to children living close to lines with less current, using Wertheimer's wire coding approach. This finding added credibility to the hypothe-sis that magnetic fields are a factor in childhood cancer. How-ever, scientists remained puzzled because the Savitz study did not find an association between the actual measurements of fields and leukemia risk.

In 1991, Dr. John Peters of the Department of Preventative Medicine at the University of Southern California School of Medicine published a study entitled "Exposure to Residential Electric and Magnetic Fields and Risk of Childhood Leukemia."[56] As in the Wertheimer and Savitz studies, Peters also reported an association between wire coding and leukemia risk in children: children living near utility lines with the highest currents had the highest risk. Interestingly, like the Savitz study, no associa-tion between actual measurements of magnetic and electric fields and leukemia risk was seen, even though the measure-ments taken in the Peters study were more extensive than that of Savitz. The Peters group used sophisticated magnetic and electric field meters.

In discussing this puzzling result, Peters suggested two possi-ble interpretations. Firstly, even the 24-hour measurements used in his study may have been a poor approximation of long-term field exposure; it may be that the wire coding approach provided a better estimate of long-term exposure to magnetic fields. Addi-tionally, since the biologically relevant feature of electromag-netic fields was not yet established, such measurements may not have recorded the important parameters. For example, features such as abrupt changes in fields could have been more impor-tant than the actual intensities of the fields.

The Peters study also looked at the self-reported use of electrical appliances by children, and found a statistically significant association between the use of both black-and-white televisions and electric hair dryers and leukemia risk. The study concluded with the suggestion that future work incorporating new knowledge of experimental electromagnetic field bioeffects may help us understand which features of the fields relate most strongly to childhood leukemia risks.

Scientists were puzzled by certain features of these leukemia studies. Several studies found an association between leukemia risk and residing near power lines judged to have the largest currents. However, neither the Savitz or Peters studies observed a similar risk when actual measurements of the fields were used instead of wire coding. Although critics had questioned whether Wertheimer's wire coding approach was an effective indirect method of assessing magnetic fields in a child's home, researchers had confirmed that this approach was indeed effective and provided an accurate picture of a home's magnetic fields. Why then the actual measurements taken in the Savitz and Peters studies would not correlate with leukemia risk became even more intriguing.

It is interesting to note the thoughts of some of the prominent epidemiologists as reported in *Microwave News*, a New York-based newsletter that has covered the electromagnetic field controversy since 1981.[57] Scientists were intrigued by what wire coding said about electromagnetic field exposures that actual measurements did not.

They suggested a number of complicating elements. For example, the direction of the magnetic field or even the earth's magnetic field may have played a role in the results. Additionally, multiple frequencies of the basic 60 Hz (120 Hz, 180 Hz, etc.) are present in varying amounts. Other complications may have been traffic density, socioeconomic status, or contaminated drinking water produced by ground current corrosion of pipes. Savitz, who suggested the idea that contaminated drinking water may be a factor linked to leukemia risk, also stated his opinion that magnetic field exposure was the "leading candidate."[57] Savitz indicated that wire coding may have provided the best assessment of long-term exposure. Dr. Samuel Milham of the Washington State University Department of Health, another epidemiologist active in this area, believes that wire codes are stable over the long term, but actual measurements may not address the critical variables for evaluating health effects.

Wertheimer also questions whether measurements of electromagnetic fields are the most important indicator, since it is not clear what exactly should be measured. The *Microwave News* articles reporting these scientific hypotheses described some of the issues raised by Nancy Wertheimer at that time.[57] Wertheimer noted that the control groups used in these studies were not entirely free of electromagnetic field exposures. She made an analogy to the difficulty in comparing risks of lung cancer in smokers of two packs of cigarettes per day to smokers of two and a half packs per day. She postulated that the magnetic field direction may have been a more critical factor than the strength of the field, and pointed to some evidence showing homes with vertical fields had less associated cancer risk than homes with horizontal fields.

Up to this point, studies of childhood leukemia risk and power line fields had raised alarm in public circles, but remaining difficulties had stopped authorities short of action. However, a recent Swedish study has represented a major epidemiological breakthrough, not only helping to clarify the relationship between childhood leukemia and power line fields, but convincing authorities, at least in Sweden, that some action is necessary. Maria Feychting and Anders Ahlbom of the Karolinska Institute of Environmental Medicine in Stockholm designed a case-control study of childhood and adult cancer from half a million people who had lived within 300 meters of a high-voltage power line between 1960 and 1985.[58] From this well-defined population, these researchers identified individuals who had contracted cancer and selected a comparable group of individuals without the disease. Using historical records of the currents carried on the power lines near each residence in the time period prior to cancer diagnosis, the magnetic fields experienced by each individual in the past were calculated with an unprecedented accuracy.

With this more accurate estimate of past exposure, a comparison of the fields of cases and controls allowed Feychting and Ahlbom to pinpoint the relationship between cancer risk and field exposure. While some cancers showed no increased risk, children were found to be 2.7 times more likely to contract leukemia if they were exposed to average fields greater than 2 mG; a 3.8 relative risk was found for those exposed to average fields greater than 3 mG.

Here for the first time was a clear demonstration of a dose-response relationship — the higher the field, the higher the risk. This study is also the most reliable so far because it used a large population in a well-defined area where other environmental influences would not affect the results. Feychting and Ahlbom's study helped explain why Peters and Savitz had not observed a relationship between increased leukemia risks and actual electromagnetic field measurements, but did find such a relationship when the wire coding approach was used instead. The Swedes also took actual measurements of fields in the residences they studied, and found no relationship to cancer. Feychting and Ahlbom explain that calculating fields from historical information, as in their study, is a refinement of the wire coding techniques because it takes more factors, in greater detail, into consideration. Thus, taking measurements in a home does not relate well to the magnetic fields that a person was exposed to in the past, in the time period leading up to cancer diagnosis. Although the Feychting and Ahlbom results are quite similar to the original Wertheimer findings, these researchers have brought another level of confidence to the association between magnetic fields from transmission lines and leukemia in children.

Radio/Microwave Epidemiology

The epidemiological research described thus far has emphasized low-frequency fields associated with electrical currents, with the strongest interest being in the magnetic part of the electromagnetic field. We shall now consider higher-frequency radio and microwave fields.

While there are protection guidelines based on heating levels of radio- and microwaves, news stories have begun to appear with examples of public and occupational concerns over more typical, non-thermal exposures from such devices as cellular telephones and police traffic radar. Despite a history of controversy over radio/microwave exposures below heating levels,[59] these high-frequency electromagnetic waves have received less attention than power line frequencies. Observations that these higher-frequency energy fields can also affect cells at levels much weaker than previously predicted does suggest the importance of studying this question.

An example of an occupational radio/microwave epidemiological study is provided by the Polish scientist Stanislaw Szmigielski.[60] Szmigielski and his co-workers examined Polish military personnel and subdivided these individuals according to whether they were exposed to radio/microwaves on the job. This was a retrospective study that grouped the subjects by age and by number of years of exposure for analysis. The Polish scientists found a three-fold increase in the incidence of cancer in the military personnel who were occupationally exposed to radio/microwaves. Their results demonstrated a relationship of increased risk with exposure duration and showed highest risks for older subjects with the longest period of exposure. Szmigielski notes that his "findings are intriguing and disturbing for epidemiologists, medical officers, as well as for society as a whole."[60] However, he cautions that his study does not "provide certain evidence of a causative relationship between the effect and the factor investigated,"[60] and adds that a more powerful prospective study currently under way should shed more light on the relationship between radio/microwave exposure and human health.

Although there is less interest in radio/microwave epidemiology, radio/microwave safety questions have a longer history of controversy than power frequencies, and with the widespread development of technologies such as cellular telephones it is an issue that will continue to be raised.

THE RESEARCH CONTROVERSY: AN OVERVIEW

It is quite impossible in a single chapter, and perhaps even in a single volume, to review all the scientific research efforts accomplished to date with respect to the interaction of living things with weak electromagnetic energy fields. This chapter has barely scraped the surface.

We have seen in many cellular and animal experiments that weak fields can affect biological functions and processes ranging from DNA synthesis to behaviour. Scientists are at a loss to understand the basic mechanisms for these effects. The existence of these effects has only recently been generally acknowledged and indeed, a few scientists still maintain that because of certain theoretical objections these results may be "artifacts" of the experimental process rather than "real" effects. These objectors are increasingly in the minority, and the search goes on for the weak field *modus operandi* that will explain these surprising, and disquieting, results. Meanwhile, many epidemiological studies have also been carried out, in both residential and occupational settings, and positive associations between serious illnesses and electromagnetic fields have been observed.

As a result, attitudes towards these various investigations are changing. A U.S. Congress Office of Technology Assessment report prepared by scientists at Carnegie-Mellon University's Department of Engineering and Public Policy in 1989 suggested that recent epidemiologic studies, although preliminary, are beginning to establish a basis for concern about possible risks from long-term exposures to electromagnetic fields. "As recently as a few years ago, scientists were making categorical statements that on the basis of all available evidence there are no health risks from human exposure to power frequency fields," the Carnegie-Mellon study stated. "In our view the emerging evidence no longer allows one to categorically assert that there are no risks."[61] And in a 1991 Electric Power Research Institute report entitled "Electric and Magnetic Field Research," it was noted that $15 million a year was being spent on research, and that

> *The ramp-up in international research mirrors a growing public concern that has been given a sharp edge of urgency by recent coverage in the popular media. While the tone is certainly more subdued in the technical literature, changes in viewpoint regarding [low-frequency fields] are also cropping up among members of the research community.*[61]

It is epidemiological research on environmental fields, particularly in the low-frequency region, that has gained the most attention and provoked heated controversy. Epidemiological research is stuck in the grey area between association and causation. While many studies have demonstrated an association between electromagnetic fields and human ill-health, the debate is over whether this association is strong enough to reflect a causal relationship. One Environmental Protection Agency committee in 1990 did go as far as to suggest a causal relationship between low-frequency magnetic fields and cancer; however, its conclusions were overruled. Some scientists maintain that other hidden factors may be the true cause of the positive associations seen in an increasing number of studies, despite the fact that even with considerable effort none have been found.

There are concerns over the lack of a clear mechanism relating electromagnetic fields to illnesses such as cancer, although many hypotheses are emerging. Many scientists are uncomfortable with some strange aspects of observed weak-field bioeffects — for example, the notion, discussed earlier, of "windows". And theoretical prejudices against the very idea of bioeffects from weak fields still linger in the scientific community. As pointed out by a Washington State Task Force on electromagnetic field reduction, many responsible scientists feel that a true relationship with human ill-health exists, while other equally responsible scientists continue to believe that future studies will not verify such a relationship.

It should not be surprising that this subject is so controversial. Epidemiological associations that are obvious today were once the subject of much debate. Smoking, for example, was until quite recently a pastime enjoyed by most adults; cigarette advertisements even featured medical doctors draped in their characteristic white lab coats enticing the public to join in the pleasure of their particular brand. When epidemiological studies began to suggest that the dangers of cigarette smoking were significant and that a public campaign should be mounted to halt the observed increase in lung cancer, the notion that tobacco was the cause of this increase was attacked. Consider, for example, the article "Alleged Dangers of Cigarette-Smoking," published in 1959 by Sir Ronald A. Fisher.[62] Fisher felt it was folly to cause anxiety amongst the public by pointing to cigarettes as the cause of an increase in lung cancer, when cigarettes may be "an entirely imaginary cause." While mounting epidemiological evidence clearly pointed to tobacco, Fisher felt that the case was by no means closed, and many scientists agreed with him. He pointed to many inconsistencies in the data at that time (related to inhalers and non-inhalers as well as pipe and cigar smokers; for example, Fisher interpreted the data as showing that inhalers got fewer cancers than non-inhalers, something that did not sit very well for the smoking-lung cancer hypothesis) which did not allow him to jump from association to causation. Fisher used an example of the correlation between an increase in apple imports and an increase in the number of divorces in Great Britain, stating that no one could conclude that one caused the other. Fisher argued that the apparent association between smoking and lung cancer could be explained by genetic differences.

Of course, Fisher's diatribe has passed into the annals of epidemiological science, and smoking is now widely recognized (except by the tobacco industry) as a causative agent for lung cancer and other illnesses. Interestingly, the number of medical doctors using tobacco declined during this period of debate, and so did their incidence of lung cancer, helping to confirm the move from association to causation. More recently debate has focused on the health hazards of second-hand cigarette smoke.

This anecdote illustrates that debate is an essential and healthy part of epidemiological research, and that proof of causality is more difficult to establish than one might first expect. Let us now explore another exciting and heated facet of scientific investigation: the search for an understanding of how unexplainable observations come about.

CHAPTER 3 NOTES

1. Gould, S.J. (1985) "Nasty Little Facts." *Natural History* February.

2. This is not to imply a conspiracy. Rather, bias is part of the process of making sense of the world in the context of scientific theories. Of course, when one considers the "experts" who are paid large sums to testify or do literature reviews for special interests, it is hard to imagine that no bias is created by this influence.

3. It has been estimated that there are up to 10,000 published reports describing studies of the interaction of non-ionizing electromagnetic fields with biological systems.

4. Most epidemiological studies to date have used exposure surrogates rather than actual measurements. For example, workers have been grouped as either exposed or not exposed to fields only by noting their job description. An assumption was made for the fields that would have been encountered in each job.

5. Liboff, A.R., T. William, D.M. Strong and R. Wistar (1984) "Time Varying Magnetic Effects on DNA Synthesis." *Science* 223, 818-820.

6. Calcium is important in many biochemical and physiological processes. For example, it plays a role in the function of muscle tissue, the hormonal action on organs such as the heart and bladder involve calcium, and the physical properties of cell membranes are affected by

calcium binding. This is in addition to its role in the functioning of the nervous system.

7. Phillips J.L., L. Rutledge and W. Winters (1986) "Transferrin Binding to Two Human Colon Carcinoma Cell Lines: Characterization and Effect of 60Hz Electromagnetic Fields." *Cancer Research* 46, 239-244.

Phillips, J.L., W. Winters and L. Rutledge (1986) "*In Vitro* Exposure to Electromagnetic Fields: Changes in Tumour Cell Properties." *International Journal of Radiation Biology* 49, 436-469.

8. Byus, C.V., K. Kartun, S. Pieper and W.R. Adey (1988) "Increased Ornithine Decarboxylase Activity in Cultured Cells Exposed to Low Energy Modulated Microwave Fields and Phorbol Ester Tumour Promoters." *Cancer Research* 48, 4222-4226.

9. Lyle, D.B., R.D. Ayotte, A.R. Sheppard and W.R. Adey (1988) "Suppression of T-Lymphocyte Cytotoxicity Following Exposure to 60 Hz Sinusoidal Electric Fields." *Bioelectromagnetics* 9, 303-313.

10. Walleczek, J. (1992) "The Immune System and ELF Electromagnetic Fields." *Frontier Perspectives* 3:1, 7-10.

11. Goodman, R. and A. Shirley-Henderson (1990) "Exposure of Cells to Extremely Low Frequency Electromagnetic Fields: Relationship to Malignancy?" *Cancer Cells* 2:11.

Goodman, R. and A. Shirley-Henderson (1991) "Transcription and Translation in Cells Exposed to Extremely Low Frequency Electromagnetic Fields." *Biochemistry and Bioenergetics* 25, 335-355.

12. Amplitude modulation of radio waves has its most common application in AM radio. A high-frequency (radio) wave is used to carry low-frequency "information" by changing (modulating) the amplitude of the carrier wave. You can think of AM radio as a low-frequency wave "mixed" in with a higher-frequency radio wave. The radio is a device which can receive the radio wave signal, "unmix" the low-frequency information and send it to a speaker. The radio wave is only needed to send the information from the radio station's transmitter to your radio. Cells and tissues also seem to have some ability to unmix an AM radio wave and respond to the low-frequency information.

13. Blackman, C.F., S.G. Benane, W.T. Jones, M.A. Hollis and D.E. House (1980) "Calcium Ion Efflux From Brain Tissue: Power Density Versus Internal Field Intensity Dependencies at 50 MHz RF Radiation." *Bioelectromagnetics* 1, 277-283.

14. Blackman, C.F., S.G. Benane, J.R.Rabinowitz, D.E. House and W.T. Jones (1985) "A Role for the Magnetic Field in the Radiation-Induced Efflux of Calcium Ions from Brain Tissue, *In Vitro*." *Bioelectromagnetics* 6, 327-337.

15. Blackman, C.F., D.E. House, G. Shawnee, S.G. Benane, W.T. Jones

and R.J. Spiegel (1988) "Effect of Ambient Levels of Power-Line-Frequency Electric Fields on a Developing Vertebrate." *Bioelectromagnetics* 9, 129-140.

16. Dutta, S.K., B. Ghosh and C.F Blackman (1989) "Radiofrequency Radiation Induced Calcium Ion Efflux Enhancement from Human and Other Neuroblastoma Cells in Culture." *Bioelectromagnetics* 10, 197-202.

17. Blackman, C.F., S.G. Benane, D.E. House and D.J. Elliott (1990) "Importance of Alignment Between Local DC Magnetic Field and an Oscillating Magnetic Field in Response of Brain Tissue *In Vitro* and *In Vivo*." *Bioelectromagnetics* 11, 159-167.

18. Blackman, C.F., S.G. Benane and D.E. House (1991) "The Influence of Temperature During Electric and Magnetic Induced Alteration of Calcium Ion Release From *In Vitro* Brain Tissue." *Bioelectromagnetics* 12, 173-182.

19. Personal correspondence with the authors (1992).

20. Adey, W.R. (1990) "Joint Actions of Environmental Non-Ionizing Electromagnetic Fields and Chemical Pollution in Cancer Promotion." *Environmental Health Perspectives* 86, 297-305.

21. The reader is referred to Adey's own research reviews for a detailed presentation of his work. The material in this book does not constitute an authoritative review; rather, we have attempted to provide some interesting examples of his research.

22. Bawin, S.M. and W.R. Adey (1976) "Sensitivity of Calcium Binding in Cerebral Tissue to Weak Environmental Electric Fields Oscillating at Low Frequency." *Proc. Nat. Acad. Sci. USA* 73:6, 1999-2003.

23. Adey, W.R. (1981) "Tissue Interactions with Non-Ionizing Electromagnetic Fields." *Physiological Reviews* 61:2, 435-511.

24. Luben, R.A., C.D. Cain, M. Chen, D.M. Rosen and W.R. Adey (1982) "Effects of Electromagnetic Stimuli on Bone and Bone Cells *In Vitro*: Inhibition of Responses to Parathyroid Hormone by Low-Energy Low-Frequency Fields." *Proc. Nat. Acad. Sci. USA* 79, 4180-4184.

25. Adey, W.R. (1987) "Evidence for Tissue Interactions With Microwave and Other Nonionizing Electromagnetic Fields in Cancer Promotion." In Fiala, J., and J. Pokorny, eds. *The Biophysics of Cancer*. Prague: Charles University, 142-151.

26. Adey, W.R. (1988) "Biological Effects of Radio Frequency Electromagnetic Radiation." In Lin, J.C. *Interaction of Electromagnetic Waves with Biological Systems*. New York: Plenum Press.

27. Vasquez, B.J., L.E. Anderson, C.I. Lowery and W.R. Adey (1988) "Diurnal Patterns in Brain Biogenic Amines of Rats Exposed to 60-Hz Electric Fields." *Bioelectromagnetics* 9, 229-236.

28. Byus, C.V., S.E. Pieper and W.R. Adey (1987) "The Effects of Low

Energy 60Hz Environmental Electromagnetic Fields Upon the Growth-Related Enzyme Ornithine Decarboxylase." *Carcinogenesis* 8:10, 1385-1389.

29. Ethical considerations for the use of animals in science are changing in response to concerns over the treatment of animals in the laboratory. The issue of animal rights continues to be debated and scientific attitudes towards the use of animals are responding in some ways to this concern.

30. Bierbaum, P.J., and J.M. Peters, eds. (1991) *Proceedings of the Scientific Workshop on the Health Effects of Electric and Magnetic Fields on Workers*, held by the National Institute of Occupational Safety and Health in Cincinnati. NIOSH Publication No. 91-111.

31. Heating damage from electromagnetic energy fields was felt to be the major consideration for human safety. Heating is only important for radio/microwaves and not lower-frequency energy fields. If adverse health effects occurred from lower-frequency fields it was felt that this should be related to the electrical currents created in the body by the fields. The strong electric fields near high-voltage power lines were thought to be a prime candidate for any possible effects. Thus, because they could create the largest electrical currents in people, most early experiments looked at effects from strong electric fields. Since the mid 1980s, much of the interest has switched to the magnetic component of the low-frequency energy fields.

32. Marino, A.A., M. Reichmanis, R.O. Becker, B. Ullrich and J.M. Cullen (1980) "Power Frequency Electric Field Induces Biological Changes in Successive Generations of Mice." *Experientia* 36, 309-311.

33. Gavalas-Medici, R. and S.R. Day-Magdaleno (1976) "Extremely Low Frequency, Weak Electric Fields Affect Schedule-Controlled Behaviour of Monkeys." *Nature* 261, 256-258.

34. Mizushima, Y., I. Akaoka and Y. Nishida (1975) "Effects of Magnetic Fields on Inflammation." *Experientia* 31, 1411-1413.

35. Circadian (daily) rhythms can demonstrate dysfunction if the length of the rhythm is altered, if the peak of a particular cycle occurs at the wrong time, or if the many different cycles lose their proper timing relative to each other.

36. Sulzman, F.M. and D.E. Murrish (1987) "Effects of Electromagnetic Fields on Primate Circadian Rhythms." In *Report of the New York State Power Lines Project*. Albany, New York: Waddsworth Centre for Laboratories and Research.

37. Wilson, B.W., E.K. Chess, L.E. Anderson (1986) "60 Hz Electric Field Effects on Pineal Melatonin Rhythms: Time Course for Onset and Recovery." *Bioelectromagnetics* 7, 239-242.

38. Oclese, J., S. Reuss and L. Vollrath (1985) "Evidence for the Involvement of the Visual System in Mediating Magnetic Field Effects on Pineal Melatonin Synthesis in the Rat." *Brain Research* 333, 382-384.

39. Salzinger, K., S. Freimark, M. McCullough, D. Phillips and L. Birenbaum (1990) "Altered Operant Behaviour of Adult Rats After Perinatal Exposure to a 60 Hz Electromagnetic Field." *Bioelectromagnetics* 11, 105-116.

40. Delgado, J.M.R., L. Jocelyne, J.L. Monteagudo and M.G. Gracia (1982) "Embryological Changes Induced by Weak, Extremely Low Frequency Electromagnetic Fields." *Journal of Anatomy* 134, 533-555.

41. Berman, E., L. Chacon, D. House, B.A. Koch, J. Leal, S. Lootrup, E. Mantiply, A.H. Martin, G.I. Martucci, K.H. Mild, J.C. Monahan, M. Sanstrom, K. Shamisaifar, R. Tell, M.A. Trillo, A. Ubeda and P. Wagner (1990) "Development of Chicken Embryos in a Pulsed Magnetic Field." *Bioelectromagnetics* 11, 169-187.

42. Cleary, S.F. (1990) "Biological Effects of Radiofrequency Radiation: An Overview." In Franceschetti, G., O.P. Gandhi and M. Grandolfo, eds. *Electromagnetic Biointeraction: Mechanisms, Safety Standards, Protection Guides*. New York: Plenum Press.

43. *Microwave News* (1990) 10:4.

44. The odds ratio (OR) can be used as an example of how such indicators are calculated. Two groups of people, exposed and not exposed to a given factor, can be further divided into groups with and those without a certain disease. Thus, four different categories are the result: P1 = exposed with the disease, P2 = exposed and without the disease, P3 = not exposed and with the disease, and P4 = not exposed and without the disease. The odds ratio is thus calculated by a ratio of ratios, (P1/P2)/(P3/P4) — that is, the ratio of disease to no disease among the exposed group divided by the ratio of disease to no disease among the non-exposed group.

45. Recall that amplitude and frequency windows describe the fact that certain frequencies create bioeffects while others do not. Additionally, biological responses, in some experiments, may only be seen within a range of intensity; either decreasing or increasing the intensity from this region will remove any observed effect. Calcium efflux experiments and Delgado's chicken egg research were examples of window observations mentioned earlier.

46. The reader is referred to the following references for more information:

Smith, C.W., R.Y.S. Choy, and J.A. Monro (1990) "The Diagnosis and Therapy of Electrical Hypersensitivities." *Journal of Clinical Ecology* 6:4, 119-128.

Rea, W.J., Y. Pan, E.J. Fenyvas, I. Sujisawa, H. Suyama, N. Samadi and G. Ross (1991) "Electromagnetic Field Sensitivity." *Journal of Bioelectricity.* 10:1-2, 241-256.

47. Much of this information was taken from the following:
Theriault, G.P. (1991) "Health Effects of Electromagnetic Radiation on Workers: Epidemiologic Studies." In Bierbaum, P.J., and J.M. Peters, eds. *Proceedings of the Scientific Workshop on the Health Effects of Electric and Magnetic Fields on Workers,* held by the National Institute of Occupational Safety and Health in Cincinnati. NIOSH Publication No. 91-111.

The reader is referred to the explicit references in this document, some 63 of which are listed. The reader is also referred to:
Electric Power Research Institute (EPRI) (1990) "Electric and Magnetic Field Research." January/February.

Ahlbom, A., E.N. Albert, A.C. Fraser-Smith, A.J. Grodzinsky, M.T. Marron, A.O. Martin, M.A. Persinger, M.L. Shelanski, and E.R. Wolpow (1987) "Biological Effects of Power Line Fields." In *Scientific Advisory Panel Final Report.* New York: New York State Power Lines Project (NYSPLP).

48. Theriault, G.P. (1991) "Health Effects of Electromagnetic Radiation on Workers: Epidemiologic Studies." In Bierbaum, P.J., and J.M. Peters, eds. *Proceedings of the Scientific Workshop on the Health Effects of Electric and Magnetic Fields on Workers.* National Institute of Occupational Safety and Health (NIOSH) Publication No. 91-111.

49. Matanowski, G. (1989) "The Hopkins Telephone and Worker Study." *Health and Safety Report* 7, 3-4.

50. Wilson, W.B. (1988) "Chronic Exposure to ELF Fields May Induce Depression." *Bioelectromagnetics.* 9, 196-205.

51. Ahlbom, A., E.N. Albert, A.C. Fraser-Smith, A.J. Grodzinsky, M.T. Marron, A.O. Martin, M.A. Persinger, M.C. Shelanski and E.R. Wolpow (1978) "Biological Effects of Power Line Fields." In *Scientific Advisory Panel Final Report.* New York: New York State Power Lines Project, 82.

52. Wertheimer, N. and E. Leeper (1986) "Possible Effects of Electric Blankets and Heated Waterbeds on Fetal Development." *Bioelectromagnetics* 7, 13-22.

53. Lindbohm, M.L., M. Hietanen, P. Kyyronen, M. Sallmen, P. Nandelstadh, H. Taskinen, M. Pekkarinen, M. Ylikoski and K. Hemminki (1992) "Magnetic Fields of Video Display Terminals and Spontaneous Abortion." *American Journal of Epidemiology* 136:9, 1041-1051.

54. In order to provide an assessment of magnetic field exposure, Wertheimer and Leeper estimated the amount of current in the electrical power line(s) near a child's home. This approach was used because

magnetic fields are related to current as opposed to voltage. This strategy, known as wire coding, was used because of the problems associated with taking and interpreting magnetic field measurements.

55. One important aspect of epidemiological research is that of confounders. Confounders are factors that may be associated with those used in the study and may be a true cause of an observed positive correlation. An example best illustrates this point. Suppose a study showed that people living in blue houses were more likely to die of liver disease. Although we may jump to the conclusion that the colour blue is hazardous to our health, it may be that a chemical pigment is present in the blue paint that has a detrimental effect on the liver and the colour blue is not directly associated with the disease. Using an example from electromagnetic field epidemiology, electrical workers may experience chemicals associated with wiring, and it is possible that the chemicals and not electromagnetic fields are the true cause of any observed positive associations. Confounders are one reason why epidemiological studies must be carefully designed and are often open to criticism. In electromagnetic field epidemiology the electromagnetic fields themselves remain the strongest candidate for an explanation of the results.

56. London, S.J., D.C. Thomas, J.D. Bowman, E. Sobel, T.C. Cheng and J.M. Peters (1991) "Exposure to Residential Electric and Magnetic Fields and Risk of Childhood Leukemia." *American Journal of Epidemiology* 134:9, 923-937.

57. *Microwave News* (1991) 11:6, 11:2.

58. Feychting, M. and A. Ahlbom (1992) "Magnetic fields and cancer in people residing near Swedish high voltage power lines." *IMM-rapport 6/92*. Sweden: Institutet för miljömedicin, Karolinska Institutet.

59. Readers interested in the controversy over radio and microwave fields will find a discussion of this in Smith, C.W. and S. Best (1989) *Electromagnetic Man: Health and Hazard in the Electrical Environment.* New York: St. Martin's Press.

60. Szmigielski, S. *et al.* (1988) "Immunologic Response to Low-Level Microwave and Radio Frequency Fields." In Marino, A.A., ed. *Modern Bioelectricity.* New York: Marcel Decker Inc., 864.

61. As quoted in: "Electric and Magnetic Field Research." *EPRI Journal*, January/February 1990.

62. Fisher, R.A. (1959) *Smoking: The Cancer Controversy.* Edinburgh: Oliver and Boyd.

FOUR

THE CHALLENGE OF A NEW FRONTIER

The most exciting challenge facing bioelectromagnetics scientists is the search to explain experiments that demonstrate an interaction between weak electromagnetic energy fields and biological systems. In the last chapter we looked at some of the changes that have been observed in cells and animals as a result of electromagnetic field exposure. This chapter will explore the present scientific framework — which does not predict such effects. In fact, some scientists even suggest outright that these effects should not occur. This discussion will lead into a presentation of a few of the many new ideas that have been proposed to provide an explanation.

The current inability to explain the *modus operandi* of weak energy fields is also a major stumbling block for progress in epidemiological research. A better insight into the nature of electromagnetic field bioeffects will greatly assist in the effort to more precisely define risks to human health. As epidemiologists learn more about which elements of these fields are critical to biological systems, their research will be better able to evaluate how the different types and levels of electromagnetic fields affect human health.

In order to introduce to the reader the scientific framework within which the debate over electromagnetic fields is taking place, this chapter will begin with a discussion of the basic concepts of electric and magnetic fields, and the electromagnetic wave and spectrum. This will lead into a discussion of the two important groupings of electromagnetic energy — ionizing and non-ionizing. The basic elements of the biointeraction of the non-ionizing electromagnetic energy fields which are the subject of this book will help to frame the controversy. As the essential background on what we do know about electromagnetic energy is sketched out, the focus of this chapter will emerge: namely, an exploration of the ideas of the frontier scientists who are working to uncover why electromagnetic fields can do what they now seem to be able to do.

THE PHYSICS OF ELECTRICITY AND MAGNETISM

Understanding the different dimensions of the electromagnetic field and health controversy is challenging. This subject involves biomedical science, epidemiology, and biology, as well as the physics of electromagnetism. This multidisciplinary nature has affected the pace of research, since the highly specialized nature of the training scientists undergo to some extent limits their ability to tackle a highly complex problem which requires a broad perspective.

An example of this difficulty was provided by Dr. Robert Becker, a researcher in the field of bioelectromagnetism. In his book *The Body Electric*, Becker commented on the difficulty in discussing the electrical properties of bone at a scientific meeting: "The engineers and physicists knew all about electronics but nothing about bone, the biologists knew all about bone but nothing about electronics and the physicians were only interested in therapeutic applications."[1] On that note, let us introduce some of the basic concepts of electromagnetism.

Electric Fields

The electric field is a concept related to the idea of force. Two like charges will repel each other while unlike charges will attract. Even though these two charges are not in direct contact, each is somehow able to affect the other. This suggests that each charge exerts a force on the other. This "action at a distance" is accomplished by virtue of a force field in space surrounding each charge. The electric field expresses the fact that at any point in this space, a second charge will experience a force. The strength of this force will be equal to the size of its charge multiplied by the size of the electric field created by the first charge. Electric fields also have directions: the electric field that sur-

TABLE 2

60 Hz ELECTRIC FIELDS AT A 30 cm DISTANCE
FROM 115V APPLIANCES*

APPLIANCE	ELECTRIC FIELD (V/m)
Electric blanket	250
Broiler	130
Stereo	90
Refrigerator	60
Electric iron	60
Hand mixer	50
Toaster	40
Hair dryer	40
Colour television	30
Vacuum cleaner	16
Incandescent light	2

* Adapted from the 1984 World Health Organization report: *Environmental Health Criteria 35, Extremely Low Frequency Fields.*

rounds a positive charge will point outward, that from a negative charge is directed inward.

An electrical conductor can produce an electric field even when there is no current flowing in the conductor. This means that electrical devices can produce electric fields even when they are not turned on.[2] This is because the electric field is related to the presence of charges in the wires; it does not matter whether these charges are actually moving (*i.e.*, whether there is a current present).

One way electric fields can be measured is in newtons per coulomb (N/C), which expresses the connection of electric fields to a force (forces are measured in newtons, and a coulomb is the unit of charge). But the measure that's more commonly used is the volt per meter (V/m) or a kilovolt per meter (kV/m, where 1 kV is equivalent to 1,000 volts). Environmental electric fields range from 40 V/m for a common appliance like a toaster, to the thousands of V/m of transmission lines (see Table 2).

The actual electric field produced by a power line will depend on a number of factors such as the height of the line, geometry and proximity of objects (buildings, trees etc.), as well as the voltage. High-voltage transmission lines will create larger electric fields than the lines associated with the lower-voltage distribution networks. Our 60 Hz electrical systems and devices produce electric fields. The term "60 Hz" means that the polarity of the electrical voltage reverses direction 60 times per second. The electric fields from 60 Hz appliances change direction in tune with the changing electrical voltage. A 60 Hz current is classified as an extra low frequency, and the fields associated with it are called extra low frequency (ELF) fields.

Electric fields are affected when you place an object within the field. A field will not penetrate the human body; rather, it will induce smaller electrical fields within us. A lot of attention has been given to the problem of calculating the fields created inside the body and electrical currents produced in animals and man from exposure to external electric fields. This has turned out to be a difficult problem.[3]

Electric fields can be reduced by shielding them with a grounded conducting surface. For example, computer screens that are grounded conductors are available; such screens reduce the electric fields that the computer operator experiences. And people working around high electric fields can wear special suits that reduce field exposure.

Until the mid 1980s, it was believed that the strong electric fields of transmission lines and substation environments were of most concern for human health. Health effects from low-frequency electromagnetic fields were expected to be related to the currents induced in the body by the fields and not directly from either the magnetic or electric components of the fields. In many types of environmental electromagnetic field exposures the largest induced currents would occur from strong electric fields. But as research during the later 1980s continued, the interest shifted away from induced currents to the magnetic component of the electromagnetic field.

Magnetic Fields

A simple example of a magnetic field is the bar magnet. This type of magnet is said to produce a "static" magnetic field, because the field does not change over time. Magnetic fields are related to charges that are moving (currents). It may not be obvious that the magnetic field from a bar magnet has a connection to the movement of an electric charge; in fact, the circulation of electrons (negatively charged particles) in their atomic orbitals are responsible for this type of magnetism.[4]

Any wire or electrical appliance with a flow of electrons (*i.e.,* electrical current) will have an associated magnetic field. The magnetic field will follow the pattern of the current. A direct current (DC) with a flow of electrons in one direction gives rise to a static magnetic field. An alternating current (AC), like the 60 Hz current in our homes, will produce magnetic fields that change in direction sixty times per second.

High school physics students are taught a trick to determine the direction of the magnetic field surrounding a wire carrying a direct current. If you grip the wire so that the thumb of your right hand points in the direction the current is flowing, your curled fingers will trace the circular pattern of the magnetic field. If you can imagine switching your grip on the wire so your thumb points in the opposing direction 60 times per second, you get a sense of what the magnetic fields surrounding a home's wiring and appliances are doing. Higher frequencies, called harmonics, may also be present in varying amounts in the electrical system. Frequencies of 120 Hz, 180 Hz, 240 Hz and other multiples of the fundamental frequency of 60 Hz may be present in the magnetic fields.

It is a quantity called the magnetic flux density (assigned the letter B) that is usually measured when environmental low-frequency magnetic fields are discussed.[5] For scientists, the preferred unit of the magnetic flux is the tesla (T). More commonly though, a unit called the gauss (G) is used, where 10,000 gauss make up one tesla. Since the fields from power lines and other environmental sources are usually even smaller than one gauss, the unit of milligauss (mG), which is one thousandth of one gauss, is most convenient to use. The 60 Hz magnetic fields produced in our homes from nearby power lines and electrical wiring typically have values of around 1 mG.

The strength of the magnetic field surrounding a current-carrying wire depends directly on the size of the current. Thus, power lines carrying high currents will be associated with correspondingly high magnetic fields. In fact, recall from Chapter 3 that some studies of childhood leukemia have used a rating of the current in the power lines near the children's homes (wire coding) rather than field measurements. Magnetic fields produced by current-carrying wires will decrease in strength with distance from the wires. It is often useful to know just how quickly these fields will decrease for a particular case. This information will help to provide an idea of how far from power lines, transformers and electrical devices the magnetic field will extend before being reduced to the background level. Often electrical appliances, such as an electric stove, will have large fields nearby, but these fields decrease rapidly with distance to background levels. An electric stove, for example, may have readings of 70 mG at 5 cm from a burner but only 1 mG at a distance of 81 cm.

Electrical wires and devices can have different magnetic field drop-off factors. This can be expressed in relation to the distance r from the device. Many household appliances will have a fall-off factor of $1/r^3$. This means that if a field of 8 mG was measured at 1 cm from a device, at 2 cm the field would already be reduced to 1 mG, and at 10 cm the field would be 0.008 mG. The magnetic field from properly paired wires (with equal and opposite current flow) will fall off at $1/r^2$, which means that an 8 mG field at 1 cm will be 2 mG at 2 cm and 0.08 mG at 10 cm. Wires in homes may also have associated fields that fall off more slowly, at a rate of $1/r$. This can occur if currents are not equal (balanced) in the two wires. In this case an 8 mG field will only fall to 4 mG at 2 cm and to 0.8 mG at 10 cm.

Magnetic fields from the distribution networks that provide electricity to our homes may decrease more slowly than magnetic fields from appliances, so that the magnetic fields will extend to greater distances before being significantly reduced. The magnetic fields from power lines are often calculated using computer programs since many complicating factors may be involved.

The direction of the magnetic field near a wire depends on the direction of the current. This can be demonstrated by the right-hand thumb rule, described above. Electrical wiring is usually done in pairs with the current in each wire opposite to that of the other. This means that the wires produce magnetic fields in opposite directions which will cancel each other out. Proper pairing of electrical wiring will keep magnetic fields as low as possible.

Power lines may have more than two wires, often called phases, but the cancellation idea still holds. In a balanced three-phase power line, the flow of current in each of the three wires is set up such that considerable magnetic field cancellation takes place. Other factors, such as the geometrical arrangement and number of wires, are also important in determining the amount of cancellation that will occur. Power utilities are currently experimenting with various field cancellation techniques to develop power lines with reduced magnetic fields.

Unlike electric fields, magnetic fields are quite difficult to shield, and low-frequency magnetic fields will penetrate the body. They are not significantly reduced by iron or lead as is sometimes believed. A special alloy called mu metal can be used to reduce the fields, but if shields are applied incorrectly, the fields can actually increase in intensity. Successful shielding requires consideration of the frequency and intensity of the magnetic fields to be shielded, and according to technicians and engineers working in this area is such a tricky business that it borders on an art form.

The Electromagnetic Wave

Electricity was first explored as long ago as 600 BC, when Thales of Miletus found that by rubbing a piece of amber, he could attract straw. The study of magnetism dates back a long time as well. The first observations of magnetism were that pieces of the natural magnetic stone magnetite (also called lodestone) would attract iron. The word magnetism comes from the name of one of the places where magnetite stones were found, Magnesia in Asia Minor.

For a long time, people studied electricity and magnetism separately without realizing there was a connection between them. In the 1820s, Hans Christian Oersted demonstrated a relationship between electricity and magnetism when he discovered that an electric current in a wire can affect a magnetic compass needle. This discovery led to some of the most important developments of 19th century physics as scientists explored the relationship between electricity and magnetism. During this time, the abstract mathematical concept of a field was used to describe experimental observations and set down fundamental physical principles. By the mid 1880s, James Clerk Maxwell was able to articulate the laws of electromagnetism. Maxwell's famous equations stand today as a pillar of the physics of electromagnetism, describing electric fields, magnetic fields and the connection between them.[6]

Electric and magnetic fields have an interesting relationship to one another: a changing magnetic field will produce an electric field, while a changing electric field will produce a magnetic field. This reciprocal relationship suggested to Maxwell that these mutually dependent oscillating fields could propagate in space as a wave.[7] The speed of this wave (the speed of light — an electromagnetic wave) can be calculated from universal constants. Since the speed is constant for a given medium, and since the frequency of any wave multiplied by its wavelength equals its speed, longer waves have smaller frequencies.

In the low-frequency region the wavelengths are so long (for example, 5000 Km at 60 Hz) that the electric and magnetic field components have to be considered independently. At higher frequencies and shorter wavelengths there is a precise relationship between the electric and magnetic fields of the wave (except for the region very close to the source); for shorter waves, electric and magnetic fields do not have to be measured independently. Instead, the energy or power of the wave can be evaluated.

These propagating electromagnetic waves can radiate outwards from a source, giving the name *electromagnetic radiation* to these waves. The word radiation is also applied to particles, such as electrons, that may be created in a number of different ways. For example, the radiation that reaches the earth's atmosphere from the sun is composed of both electromagnetic and particulate radiation.

Thus, at low frequencies of oscillation such as the 60 Hz of our electric power systems, electric and magnetic field components are considered separately. At higher frequencies, the precise relationship between the magnetic and electric components of the wave means that the energy or power of the electric and magnetic parts of the wave can be considered together. Radio and microwaves are often evaluated in terms of the amount of energy per unit of time per unit area (W/m^2), although reference can be made specifically to the electric and magnetic components of radio and microwaves.

In order to efficiently get the energy of electric and magnetic fields to propagate outwards as a wave, it is necessary to have an appropriate transmitting antenna. It helps for the antenna to have a size that compares to the length of the waves that are to be propagated. Radio waves can have lengths on the order of meters and the sizes of transmitting and receiving antennae reflect this scale. On the other hand if you wanted to effectively send electromagnetic waves of low frequency you would need a very big antenna (remember the 5000 km at 60 Hz). It turned out that low frequencies were useful for communications to submarines. The United States military project codenamed Sanguine (see Chapter 2) was a plan to bury an antenna in a large area of the state of Wisconsin to send electromagnetic signals to the submarine fleet.

The Electromagnetic Spectrum

The amount of energy contained in an electromagnetic wave is directly proportional to its frequency of oscillation.[8] It is the amount of energy that will determine how the wave interacts with matter, and all possible energies constitute what is called the electromagnetic spectrum. Despite the different properties of these waves, all electromagnetic waves travel at the same speed, namely the speed of light: 3.0×10^8 m/s in a vacuum.

Visible light is an electromagnetic wave which oscillates at approximately 10^{15} times a second. The actual frequency has a direct relationship to what we perceive as colours, ranging from red at lower frequencies to blue at higher frequencies. Ultraviolet (UV) waves have a slightly higher frequency than visible light, and have the ability to damage molecules. (The ozone layer which surrounds the Earth blocks most of the ultraviolet waves which bombard our planet; the concern over depletion of this ozone layer derives from the fact that more of this UV radiation is now getting through and can detrimentally affect a wide range of organisms, including humans.) Higher-frequency oscillations produce waves which are known as X-rays (around 10^{18} oscillations per second) and gamma-rays (above 10^{20} oscillations per second). These waves have the distinct property of being able to directly damage molecules.

Infrared waves have frequencies lower than that of visible light, ranging down to 10^{12} oscillations per second. Infrared waves may cause skin burns and can produce cataracts if exposure is prolonged. Ultraviolet, visible and infrared waves are often called optical radiations.

At even lower frequencies the waves become longer, ranging in length from millimeters to many hundreds of meters. Radio and microwaves are found in this region of the electromagnetic spectrum. They are used for such things as the transmission of information (communications, radio, television, etc.) and heating (microwave ovens). Even lower than radio and microwaves are the two lowest frequency regions that are called, not surprisingly, very low frequency (VLF) and extra (or extremely) low frequency (ELF). These long waves include 60 Hz, the frequency chosen for our electrical power systems, which happens to be an ELF frequency.

Radio and microwaves contain enough energy to cause heating. ELF and VLF waves contain less energy than radio and microwaves. ELF electric and magnetic fields do not have enough energy to cause heating like microwaves, although they can create currents in our bodies.

ELECTROMAGNETISM AND LIFE:
AN OUTLINE OF THE CONTROVERSY

In order to understand the background of this issue it is useful to outline the basic tenets of the current scientific ideas. Our present understanding of the relationship between electromagnetic energy and living things is the place to begin. We shall see that the observation of biological effects from weak electromagnetic energy fields does not easily fit into the current theoretical framework.

Electromagnetic energy can be divided into two types based on its effect on matter. High-frequency, short-wavelength electromagnetic waves contain a large amount of energy. This energy is able to knock electrons out of their atomic orbits, creating atoms (called ions) that have a reduced number of electrons. It is because of this ability to create ions that X-rays and gamma-rays are said to be ionizing. Together with a number of high-energy particles, these electromagnetic waves are called ionizing radiation.

Electromagnetic waves that do not have enough energy to knock electrons out of their atomic orbits are said to be non-ionizing. Non-ionizing electromagnetic energy includes visible light, microwaves, radio waves, and electromagnetic fields at very low and extra low frequencies. The controversy over power line fields, cellular phones and other environmental electromagnetic energy sources involves this lower-frequency, longer-wavelength non-ionizing category.

The biological consequences of electromagnetic energy exposures are related to the different effects these waves can have on matter. X-rays and gamma-rays can directly damage biological molecules, based on their abilities to knock electrons from molecules and atoms, and have well established effects.[9] Exposures to this type of energy are now well regulated although in the early days of X-ray technology little was known about the dangers. For example, it was not so long ago that X-rays were used in shoe stores to correctly size shoes! Scientists have continued to learn more about the effects of X-rays and other ionizing radiations on human health, and safety standards have continued to become more strict.

Thermal and Non-Thermal Effects

Non-ionizing energy fields are too weak to directly damage biological molecules. However, non-ionizing energy fields can create biological effects through the heating of tissue. Microwaves and radio waves do not have enough energy to directly ionize atoms and molecules, but they do have enough energy to cause heating. The microwave oven is based on this heating potential of microwave fields. In a microwave oven, the microwave's energy is absorbed by the food, turned into heat, and the food is cooked. Changes produced in biological organisms related to the heating ability of radio and microwave fields are called *thermal effects*. Safety limits for radio and microwaves have been developed by considering how much heating a person can tolerate before the natural thermoregulatory mechanisms of the body are overly taxed.

The thermal limit safety standard is based on research carried out in the 1950s by the scientist Herman Schwan, and is sometimes called the Schwan limit. This limit represents an estimate of how much heating the human body can withstand from radio and microwave exposure. Schwan based his estimates of heating on models of physiological systems using salt water. This limit was adopted in the 1960s as a guideline for occupational safety, and has been revised to take into account the fact that the waves are absorbed more readily when the length of the wave is comparable to the size of the human body.

Until now, scientists believed that it is important to limit our exposure to high-energy X-rays because of the direct damage these waves can do to our biological molecules, and that our exposure to radio waves and microwaves should be limited to levels below those which can cause problems related to heating in our bodies. These have been the dominant considerations for human exposure to electromagnetic energy. However, as we saw in Chapter 3, research examining the biological effects of weak electromagnetic energy fields shows there are other considerations besides ionization and heating ability. Here, "weak" means energy levels and intensities below those able to cause direct molecular damage or thermal (heating) effects.

Electromagnetic waves that have even less energy than radio or microwaves fall into the very low frequency (VLF) and extra low frequency (ELF) regions. These waves have long wavelengths and do not contain enough energy to heat matter, let alone create molecular damage. The view that this form of energy cannot possibly have effects on biological systems is now challenged by experimental results confirming that low-frequency electromagnetic energy is able to produce changes in cells, tissues and animals. There is also an increasing number of observations of bioeffects from radio and microwaves at levels below those necessary to create significant heating. Such effects on biological systems from weak non-ionizing fields have been called *non-thermal effects*, in contrast to the well established idea of heating (thermal) effects.

These basic concepts (see Figure 4) help to provide an outline of the controversy. Individuals experience a wide range of fields at non-thermal levels in their daily lives, ranging from the 60 Hz magnetic energy of their hair dryers to the higher frequency radio/microwave fields of cellular telephones. The very basic question that has provoked controversy is whether these weak non-thermal fields have the ability to produce changes in living organisms. If not, then there is no means by which the weak fields we experience in our daily lives could affect our health, adversely or otherwise. In contrast, the existence of weak field bioeffects suggest that it is indeed important to investigate human health questions, whether the sources of these fields are power lines, electric blankets or cellular telephones. The existence of non-thermal effects from weak fields does not necessar-

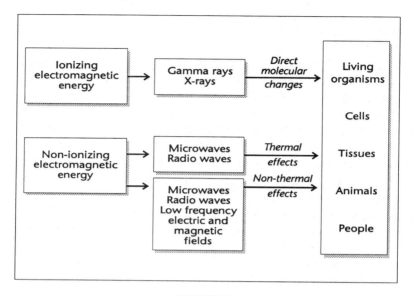

FIGURE 4

Schematic depiction of the interaction between electromagnetic energy and living organisms. The fundamental difference between ionizing and non-ionizing energy is emphasised. The controversial questions dealt with in this book involve effects from non-ionizing fields at energies and intensities below those required for heating to occur. Heating can result from higher intensities of radio and microwaves. Low frequency magnetic and electric fields are too weak to heat tissue.

ily imply adverse human health effects, although this is a closely related issue. Other related research includes the search for new medical applications and for a deepened understanding of life processes.

Within the present scientific paradigm, non-thermal effects should not exist because there is no mechanism for effects on cells or multicellular organisms at such weak energies. However, research over the last two decades indicates that such non-thermal effects do indeed exist, and so the basic paradigm is directly challenged. Even now some scientists feel that the experiments of the different research groups showing non-thermal effects are not valid, because there is no widely accepted theory to account for their findings.

Despite these objectors, there is now a change in attitude among scientists, as a result of the overwhelming number of experiments which demonstrate non-thermal effects. The debate over whether weak fields can be biologically active has a growing consensus to the affirmative. For example, even the Electric Power Research Institute (EPRI), a research body funded by power utilities, points to the growing number of examples of effects from weak fields. In a 1990 report, EPRI stated:

The biological research literature abounds with reports of [low-frequency field] effects, ranging from altered calcium ion flux across cell membranes to activation of enzymes, changes in cells' immune activity, endocrine system changes, and alteration of DNA, RNA, and protein synthesis.[10]

Echoing a similar acknowledgement of the existence of bioeffects from weak fields, a 1989 United States Office of Technology Assessment report noted, "It is now clear that 60 hertz and other low frequency electromagnetic fields can interact with individual cells and organs to produce biological changes."[11]

While the existence of non-thermal effects is now widely accepted, the problem for scientists is to explain why and how they occur. Many ideas about mechanisms for interactions of non-ionizing energy with biological systems at non-thermal intensities have been proposed, but there is, as of yet, no widely accepted explanation for how non-thermal effects occur.

There are two possible scenarios for future research. A single or multiple mechanism(s) may be discovered that falls within the current paradigm and can successfully describe the wide range of non-thermal effects now found in the peer-review scientific literature. Secondly, the observation of effects that are not easily explained give rise to an intense scrutiny of the basic assumptions underlying the current paradigm. A number of scientists are exploring novel ways of understanding the organization and communication of biological systems. The observation of unexplainable effects may well create interest in these frontier areas of research.

MECHANISMS OF INTERACTION

One of the basic problems hindering the whole field of bioelec-tromagnetics is the lack of a well-defined and generally accepted mechanism (or mechanisms) whereby these types of fields can influence biological systems. In fact, there have been a number of fundamental theoretical objections to the idea that non-ther-mal bioeffects from this type of energy even exist at all! After discussing two of those theoretical stumbling blocks for scien-tists, this section will present some of the proposed non-thermal mechanisms of interaction between non-ionizing electromag-netic energy and cells, tissue and man.

Theoretical Objections

One theoretical problem with understanding electromagnetic field bioeffects at non-thermal levels has to do with the cell membrane. The cell owes its existence to a membrane which separates it from its external environment. It uses a lot of energy to maintain the kind of internal environment required for opti-mum functioning. The membrane is an active barrier that makes this compartmentalization possible. The membrane is one of the most important parts of the cell.

An electric potential (voltage) exists across the membrane as a result of the charge difference between the outside and inside of a cell. This voltage, though small, exists over the microscopic di-mensions of the membrane, thereby producing a large electric field.[12] It has been suggested that the cell is, in a sense, protected from the influence of (smaller) external fields by this very large internal field. The electric fields induced in the body by typical environmental fields will be much smaller than the membrane field.

Another objection raised by some scientists has to do with "thermal noise". Living biological material is subject to a random thermal movement of the biological molecules. This dancing-around-and-bumping-into-each-other behaviour of molecules, called thermal noise, only ceases at absolute zero temperature (-273° C). Under most circumstances, the energy produced by this thermal noise is stronger than the energy created by low-frequency magnetic fields. Thus, another theoretical objection is that biological systems could not be affected by non-thermal electromagnetic fields because the energy they impart to a cell or tissue will be swamped by the large thermal noise energy. As a crude analogy, imagine a group of children playing in bumper cars, moving back and forth, stopping, starting and bouncing off one another. Now, imagine a housefly striking one of the carts. Clearly the fly's accident would go quite unnoticed by the children in their larger and heavier carts.

A number of arguments have been presented to overcome such objections. Firstly, the external fields created by such things as power lines are (in the vast majority of cases) alternating at particular frequencies, while the cell's large membrane field is static (DC). Comparing fields that are alternating and fundamentally different from fields that are stationary, the argument goes, is like comparing apples to oranges. Other scientists point to the evidence that electromagnetic fields play a role in some biological processes, and organisms may have evolved mechanisms to sense weak environmental fields.[13] Thus, the presence of special abilities to sense external fields even at typically weak environmental levels would make comparisons to the membrane field irrelevant.

Secondly, as scientists like Ross Adey suggest, these dismissals of weak field effects ignore the important cooperative nature of biological systems.[14] Adey points out that long-range interactions described by new developments in branches of physics such as quantum theory may provide a basis for understanding biological responses to weak electromagnetic stimuli. Adey's model proposes that electromagnetic signals are important in cellular communication and that weak external fields can be amplified by already existing mechanisms at the cell membrane, thereby interfering with cellular processes.

The problem of the thermal noise limit objection was the subject of a paper published in the prestigious journal *Science* by Drs. James Weaver and Dean Astumian.[15] Weaver and Astumian presented a physical model that overcame "the apparent violation of the thermal noise limit seen in some experiments."[15] Using mathematics, they showed that cells can indeed act as detectors of very weak fields as observed in numerous experiments. In their conclusion, Weaver and Astumian stated that the possibility of biological effects from weak environmental electromagnetic fields cannot be ignored because of the noise objection.

A further challenge to such objections is the recent discovery of magnetic material in the human brain.[16] Despite findings of magnetic magnetite in bacteria, mollusks, salmon, and honeybees, among others, humans were considered to be 100 per cent non-magnetic. The possibility of built-in human magnetic sensors suggests a sensitivity to weaker electromagnetic fields than would be otherwise expected.

Fighters deliver their jabs and blows in the boxing ring; scientists throw their punches within the forum of the scientific journal. These struggles, although intellectually based, are no less emotionally charged. A recent bout over the biological effects of weak fields took place in the journal *Physical Review*, and serves as an interesting example of the theoretical objections.[17]

Dr. Robert Adair, a Yale University physics professor, published a paper in 1991 entitled "Constraints on Biological Effects of Weak Extremely-Low-Frequency Electromagnetic Fields." Adair concluded that the interactions between weak fields and the cells within the human body are too weak to have any significant effect. He felt that "any biological effects of weak ELF fields on the cellular level must be found outside of the scope of conventional physics," thus implying the nonexistence of reported observations to the contrary. Adair's analysis proceeded from his assumption that biological interactions of weak fields must be greater than the thermal interactions of the biomolecules with their environment. This is basically a statement of the thermal noise objection. Adair calculated the energy of interaction between weak electric and magnetic fields and physical models of cells, and estimated the thermal noise present in a cell. He concluded that even for a wide assortment of interaction scenarios, weak field energies are well below the level of thermal noise and thus were constrained in their ability to produce biological changes.

In a further blow to and scathing indictment of much of bioelectromagnetics research, and in direct conflict with the conclusions of scientists active in that area, Adair states that "The experimental record lacks coherence and credibility. After 20 years of experimentation, no significant effect of weak ELF fields at the cell level has been firmly established." Adair criticised the lack of satisfactory replication of experiments that found weak field effects, and pointed to the complex and subtle nature of the effects observed as evidence of their nonexistence. He had particular trouble with the observation of "windows" and the apparent non-linear responses of biological systems to weak fields. (Scientists are much more comfortable with linear effects. If a spring stretches 1 cm when you hang a 1 Kg mass from one end, a 2 Kg mass should stretch the spring 2 cm. In contrast, in many experiments of weak fields with cells, increasing the fields will not produce a corresponding increase in the observed effect.) Since this analysis would suggest that the observations of bioelectromagnetics researchers are no more than figments of their overactive imaginations, it is not hard to see the emotional quality of such an attack.

In answer to Adair, Dr. Joseph Kirschvink, the discoverer of magnetite crystals in human brain tissue and a researcher long involved in studies of biomagnetism, published an article in a

1992 issue of *Physical Review* entitled "Comment on 'Constrains on Biological Effects of Weak Extremely-Low-Frequency Electromagnetic Fields'." In a direct counter-punch to Adair's conclusion that weak low-frequency fields could not possibly affect cells, Kirschvink bluntly stated, "Adair's assertion that few cells of higher organisms contain magnetite (Fe_3O_4) and his blanket denial of reproducible ELF effects on animals are both wrong." Adair had only considered the magnetic crystals in a particular species of bacteria for one of his calculations on weak field interactions, Kirschvink argued.

Kirschvink's rebuttal was drawn along three lines. First, he noted that humans and other organisms have magnetite in many of their body's cells, and organisms can be considered sensitive to external signals even if only a few cells respond. Further, magnetosomes (magnetite-containing structures enclosed by a membrane) may occur in chains, and there is a great similarity between those found in salmon and those first discovered in magnetotactic bacteria. Kirschvink concludes that Adair's analysis is contradicted by the fact that some higher animals can manufacture miniature magnets which allow them to strongly interact even with weak low-frequency magnetic fields.

The second part of Kirschvink's rebuttal centred on Adair's view that there are no firmly established biological effects of any significance from weak low-frequency fields. Kirschvink noted that a demonstration of weak field-induced changes in animal behaviour would be more than enough to counter Adair's claim. Because of Kirschvink's experience in working with honeybees, he elaborated the many experiments, as well as replications, investigating magnetic effects on honeybee behaviour. Kirschvink presented a table describing eight different effects on honeybee behaviour and added that, to his knowledge, all attempts to replicate these experiments were successful. He described research showing that honeybees looking for food can detect small changes in the earth's magnetic field, and noted other "simple and direct" experiments demonstrating an influence of power-frequency magnetic fields on bee behaviour. In one experiment cited by Kirschvink, a bee was able to respond to changes in the earth's field as low as 0.06 per cent of the actual geomagnetic field. Small magnetized wires attached to a bee's abdomen affected its ability to detect changes in the earth's magnetic field. Similar experiments with copper wires, which are not magnetic, had no such effects. Kirschvink concludes:

The honeybee data provide clear and reproducible evidence that at least one terrestrial animal is influenced at the cellular level by weak ELF magnetic fields. Hence, the existence of similar effects in other magnetite containing cells cannot be dismissed a priori as done by Adair.[17]

The third part of Kirschvink's reply to Adair consisted of a model that explains how weak fields could interact with biological magnetite (described later in this chapter). He summarizes with his opinion that:

[T]here are very good reasons to believe that weak ELF fields can and do have significant biological effects at the cell level, and the process of magnetite biomineralization provides at least one viable mechanism through which such things can happen. The credibility of weak ELF magnetic effects on living systems must therefore stand or fall mainly on the merits and reproducibility of the biological or epidemiological experiments which suggest them, rather than on dogma about physical implausibility.

The use of the word dogma, a verbal right hook, illustrates the paradigm-challenging nature of bioelectromagnetics! Kirschvink felt that it was wrong to reject cellular and animal low-frequency field experiments and epidemiological research simply because Adair lacked the ability to come up with a physically plausible mechanism.

Let us now explore some of the ideas that have been proposed to explain how weak fields could interact with living organisms.

Resonance Mechanisms

As we have seen, the challenge is to understand how the small amount of energy contained in weak electromagnetic energy fields could be amplified to produce physiological changes. There is in fact a well-known physical phenomenon whereby a very small signal produces a large change. This phenomenon is known as resonance. There are many examples of resonance throughout the physical sciences.

Resonance describes the interaction between a physical oscillating system and an external driving force. As a concrete example, consider a playground swing (the physical oscillating system) and your push (the external driving force). The system (swing) will have a natural frequency of motion (careful playground observers will have noticed the number of times the swing moves back and forth per second depends on the length of the swing's ropes; longer ropes mean a longer time to go back and forth). If the external driving force is applied at a frequency that matches the natural frequency of motion of the system, then resonance occurs. The external signal or force will have a maximum effect on the system. In our swing example, to get the largest back and forth motion we naturally push the swing at the same frequency as its movement; otherwise we end up wasting our effort by pushing forward while it is still moving backwards.

One widely used example of resonance is the Tacoma Narrows Bridge incident, often described in introductory physics text books. A large suspension bridge in Washington State collapsed soon after construction. The bridge had a natural resonance with the wind that blew through the Tacoma Narrows. Such large movements were created in the bridge that it literally self-destructed even though the wind was nothing more than a strong breeze.

Several resonance mechanisms have been proposed as explanations for the bioeffects that have been observed in response to weak energy fields. Nuclear magnetic resonance, electron paramagnetic resonance, and cyclotron resonance are all complex resonance phenomena, well known in physics, that have been proposed in this context. The most widely studied is that of cyclotron resonance.[18] The cyclotron resonance phenomenon may help to explain how low-frequency fields could move biologically significant ions such as calcium, sodium and lithium across channels of a cell membrane.

Cyclotron resonance refers to the motion of a charged particle in a static magnetic field. Charged particles move in a circular or elliptical path when under the influence of a stationary (static) magnetic field like that of the earth. This circular motion will have a characteristic frequency and radius of orbit which will depend on the size of the charge, the mass of the particle, and the strength of the magnetic field. If a second, alternating field is applied with a frequency that matches the frequency of the circular motion of the particle, a resonance condition will be set up. This means a particle can absorb energy most efficiently from the alternating field and its motion will be affected.

Dr. Abraham Liboff first considered cyclotron resonance as an explanation for the calcium efflux observations described in Chapter 3.[19] He suggested that the earth's static magnetic field could create a circular path with characteristic frequencies for different biologically important ions which are charged particles. For example, chlorine (Cl^-) has a single negative charge, sodium (Na^+) has a single positive charge, while calcium (Ca^{2+}) has two positive charges. The externally applied fields used in the laboratory experiments on calcium binding (or low-frequency environmental electromagnetic fields like the 60 Hz ones produced by household electricity) would be in resonance, and a lot of their energy absorbed, if their frequency matched the orbital frequency created by the earth's static field.

Liboff calculated the cyclotron frequencies that are produced by the earth's field for a number of biologically important ions (see Figure 5). He found that some frequencies were in the correct range to provide an explanation. For example, magnesium (Mg^{2+}) has a cyclotron resonance frequency of about 60 Hz at a

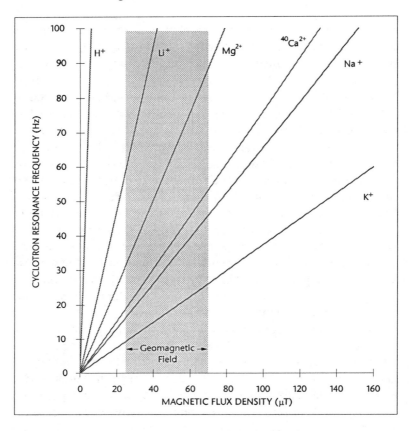

FIGURE 5

Charged particles like ions have circular orbits when they move at right-angles to a static magnetic field. If an applied alternating field has a frequency that matches the orbital frequency of the ion, then cyclotron resonance occurs. The geomagnetic field ranges from 250 to 700 mG (25 to 70 microtesla). Many biologically important ions have low-frequency cyclotron resonance for typical values of the earth's magnetic field. Adapted from: *The Cyclotron Resonance Hypothesis: An EMF Health Effects Resource Paper*, EPRI, 1990.

typical value of the earth's field. Calcium has a lower frequency, about 30 Hz for this same field. Carl Blackman's research, discussed in Chapter 3, has also contributed to the hypothesis of cyclotron resonance.

Cyclotron resonance has been a very useful concept to help explain the results of calcium efflux experiments where particular frequencies were seen to be more effective than others in influencing the binding of calcium to brain tissues. Blackman also demonstrated experimentally that the earth's static magnetic field plays a role in the influence of weak energy fields on the calcium efflux observations.

After the proposal of the cyclotron resonance hypothesis, other experiments have attempted to verify and test for this effect. For example, an experiment performed by J.R. Thomas and J. Schrot working with Liboff, studied the ability of rats to respond to lever press training under cyclotron resonance conditions for lithium ions.[20] Each animal in this study showed a clearly reproducible change in its response behaviour when the fields were applied in such a way as to produce cyclotron resonance for the lithium ion. The animals seemed to be unable to estimate the time required between pushes of a lever to release a food pellet. They pushed the lever too quickly and seemingly randomly. The scientists hypothesized that an efflux of lithium ions from cells in rat brains played a role in their observations.

However, while some experiments, like those examining rat behaviour under lithium resonance, seem to support the cyclotron hypothesis, other experiments have found no evidence of effects under calculated resonance conditions. Several theoretical problems still need to be overcome in order for the resonance model to be more widely applied. The cyclotron resonance hypothesis is part of a preliminary attempt to understand electromagnetic field bioeffects and is one mechanism for an electromagnetic field influence on the movement of ions across cell membranes.

Stress Response

Another way of looking at the relationship between electromagnetic fields and health has been proposed by the biophysicist Dr. Andrew Marino.[21] Marino views the effects of low-frequency fields on animals and humans within the context of what are known as environmental stressors. That is, chronic electromagnetic field exposure will result in a generalized stress response and hence in an increase in the many illnesses associated with a deterioration of an organism's adaptive capacity.

Marino interprets the results of studies of rodents exposed to fields in terms of a hypothesis describing a sequence of physiological changes. He feels that these changes provide evidence for a chronic stressor effect from environmental electromagnetic fields. The Marino model proposes that the fields are detected by the peripheral or central nervous system. Since there is a close relationship between the nervous, endocrine, and immune systems, a response could manifest itself in various organs and body functions.

Marino points out that extensive clinical observations implicate stressors as a risk factor for diseases such as diabetes, cancer and cardiovascular pathology. However, he is careful to note that no general theory predicts an outcome of the effect of a particular stressor on an organism — given the complexity of factors in the organism's life.

Stress-induced changes in the immune system are one possible cause of long-term health consequences from chronic exposure to a stressor. This approach suggests that since all human diseases can be affected by stressors, there are no reasons to expect particular diseases to appear as a result of electromagnetic field exposure. Thus, if there is validity to this approach, field effects on health will be non-specific and submerged within the influence of the myriad environmental, social and psychological stresses to which we are all subjected.

Marino's stressor hypothesis has not been well received in the scientific community. Researchers have criticized the data of the animal studies to which Marino refers. They describe them as being inconsistent and inconclusive. Problems in the design of these early experiments have prompted scientists to question the results and hence conclusions. General qualitative models of stressors are not satisfying to the scientific community, which expects more quantitative, mechanistic and rigorous approaches to understanding electromagnetic field bioeffects.

Marino has countered this accusation, maintaining that this early data does indeed demonstrate electromagnetic field bioeffects, the existence of which was the main contention at that stage. As has been pointed out, the relationship between smoking and lung cancer emerged long before a mechanism was suggested for carcinogenesis. The specific carcinogenic factors in cigarette smoke are still not identified, and smoking is known to be a risk factor for other illnesses such as heart disease, emphysema, and cancer of the bladder without specific mechanisms of action being well understood. Marino, in testimony before a public inquiry into power line fields, has stated that true causality in science may never be demonstrated, and inference of electromagnetic field bioeffects must be relied upon.[22]

Hormonal Changes

The pineal gland is a pinecone-shaped structure in the centre of the head. This gland produces an assortment of active biological molecules (hormones) which regulate the activity of other glands and help to regulate brain activity. Hormones produced by the pineal gland include melatonin, serotonin and dopamine, all important components of the body's chemical control system. Of particular interest is the role that these hormones play in biological rhythms. For example, the cyclic sleep/wake pattern is dependent on melatonin secreted by the pineal gland.

Two observations about this control system suggest a connection to health effects from exposure to low-frequency electromagnetic fields. Firstly, electromagnetic fields have been shown to alter daily rhythms in the levels of pineal hormones, thereby affecting circadian rhythms.[23] Secondly, changes in melatonin levels have been shown to be related to some hormonally influenced tumours, such as breast cancer. If melatonin plays a role in cancer and electromagnetic fields can influence this hormone's secretion from the pineal gland, an indirect mechanism can be postulated whereby adverse health effects could result from field exposure.

In several studies male breast cancer, a very rare disease, has been found to occur more often than expected among electrical workers.[24] A preliminary study of breast cancer in women using electric blankets did not support the hypothesis of such a connection, although it did show a small (not statistically significant) increase.[25] Nonetheless this hypothesis has captured increasing interest, and more studies investigating this connection can be expected.

To complete this hypothesis, an explanation is required to describe how low-frequency fields could affect the hormonal secretions of the pineal gland. One researcher at the University of Texas, Dr. Russel Reiter, has pointed out that abrupt changes in magnetic fields will produce currents in the eye and create the visual impression of light.[26] The brain may respond to these light signals at night by decreasing melatonin levels, which are normally elevated during the night. Rütger Wever, a German scientist researching biological rhythms, found that cues from the earth's magnetic field may be used in establishing biological rhythms in humans. This again reinforces the idea that electromagnetic fields may affect biorhythms and hints that there may be some way by which we have the ability to sense very weak fields.

A Magnetic Field-Sensing Organ

An organ capable of sensing magnetic fields would help to provide an explanation for phenomena such as weak field-induced hormonal changes, and the apparent ability of humans to use weak fields as timing cues for cyclic rhythms. In fact, small crystals of magnetite have been discovered in a wide range of living organisms including bacteria, bees, pigeons and sharks. The recent announcement by Dr. Joseph Kirschvink of the California Institute of Technology at Pasadena, that magnetite particles ranging from 50 to 600 nanometers (one nanometer is 10^{-9} meters — one billionth of a meter) in length are present in the human brain, is of great interest to bioelectromagnetics researchers.[16] Magnetite crystals are apparently manufactured in animals; Kirschvink observed that the human crystals also appear to be the result of a biological process. These human crystals were identical to those found in bacteria. The crystals were found in bunches of 50 to 100, and more than 100 million crystals were found per gram of tissue from certain parts of the brain. The role magnetic crystals may play in human physiology will undoubtedly be the focus of many future studies. Certainly, the possibility of magnetic crystals in brain tissue will present many future opportunities to understand electromagnetic field bioeffects. These magnetic particles can have over a million times stronger response to magnetic fields than normal non-magnetic tissue.

Kirschvink recently presented a preliminary model describing how low-frequency magnetic fields could create significant biological changes.[17] The model, described in Figure 6, involves channels in the cell membrane which are used to control the flow of ions into the cell. Some of these ion channels have gates that can be mechanically opened and closed. Kirschvink noted that this kind of channel is present in almost every organism and tissue. These channels need only be open for a very short period of time for the nervous system to be stimulated.

The next feature of the model is the fact that many parts of cells are known to be held in place by protein-containing filaments that are part of what is known as the cytoskeletal system. It is likely that magnetosomes have attachments to the cell membrane and the ion channel. This attachment can be thought of as a gating-spring. According to Kirschvink's model, a magnetosome under the influence of the Earth's magnetic field can be

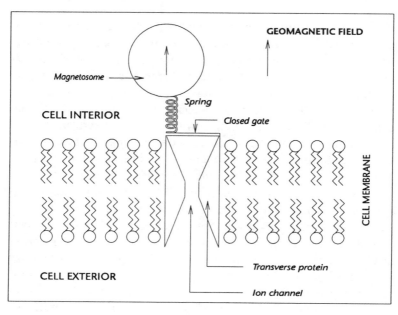

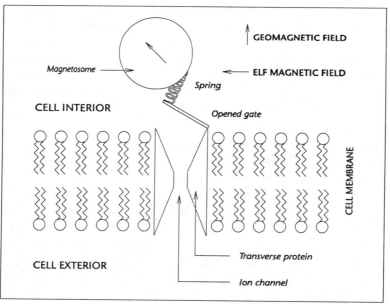

rotated by a low-frequency magnetic field, and this rotation opens the normally closed ion gate. Calculations show that the main flaw of this model is that low-frequency magnetic fields greater than the 500 mG of the geomagnetic field would be required to open the ion channels.

Cellular Communication

The work of W. Ross Adey was described in Chapter 3. Adey's model for low-frequency field effects involves a process whereby weak electromagnetic signals can directly interfere with communications from the outside of the cell to the cell interior. In this model, the influence of weak electromagnetic fields at the cell membrane can change chemical events and amplify triggers associated with the binding of important biomolecules, including hormones and neurotransmitters. Adey postulates that calcium ions play an important role in the amplification of such weak stimuli, even at levels millions of times weaker than the field of the cell membrane. Since in this model electromagnetic fields can directly interfere with intercellular communications, the action of cancer promoters that have effects on the cell membrane could be enhanced by the presence of low-frequency fields. Thus, Adey asserts that field effects on the cancer process are distinct from cancer initiation and involve the interference with normal cell-to-cell communication.[27]

FIGURE 6 (Facing Page)

Model of how a mechanically sensitive ion channel could be opened by a low-frequency magnetic field. The magnetosome should be larger than shown. A) The magnetosome is attached to the ion channel by a cytoskeletal filament which can be thought of as a gating spring. The channel is normally closed. B) A low-frequency magnetic field could interact with the magnetosome, causing it to rotate and open the gate. Ions like Ca^{2+} easily travel through these channels and in doing so can produce changes in the cell. Adapted from J.L. Kirschvink. *Phys. Rev. A.* 1992. 46:4, 2179.

New Frontiers in Physical Theory

The quantum theory has revolutionized our understanding of the physical world, and has shown that so-called classical approaches are limited. The study of biological systems, on the other hand, has remained largely within the classical domain.[28] While the quantum theory is useful for understanding how very small things like atoms, electrons and subatomic particles work, most features of larger objects, even the size of cells, can be described by the older (classical) approaches. Thus, it has been assumed that biology is "too big" for quantum-based approaches. And it has been chemistry, not physics that has played the dominant role in the development of modern biology and medicine. The ultimate discovery of contemporary biology, the gene, is a chemical and we continue to search for new drugs, chemicals, to cure disease.

While the greatest efforts of the biological and medical sciences are focused on learning more about the fundamental parts of living things, the biochemicals, basic questions are increasingly being raised about what puts it all together: just how the whole is created from the parts. It is in this area that physics may begin to play a larger role in biology. The application of non-classical physical models and the development of new physical theories in the study of biological organization and integration is a fascinating frontier of science. The scope of research in this area is broad and undefined, and the theoretical elements are quite complex. The interested reader is referred to some suggested readings in the chapter endnotes.[29]

Quantum theory and other non-classical physical theories may provide a mechanism (or mechanisms) whereby weak energy fields could influence biological organization and function. In fact, it may be that very weak electromagnetic signals play a fundamental role in biological processes through cellular communication or long-range biomolecular interaction. For example, Adey repeatedly emphasizes that the cooperative nature of biological systems (*i.e.*, how the parts of complex living systems work together) cannot be understood in terms of equilibrium thermodynamics and the classical models of statistical mechanics — the older way of doing things.[30] He suggests that to study cooperative phenomena, which are important in understanding the effects of weak electromagnetic signals, non-linear, non-equilibrium electrodynamics and quantum processes, all more recent advances in physical theory, must be utilized.

Dr. Emilio DelGuidice, an Italian researcher working to develop new approaches to understand the interaction of physical systems and keenly interested in the application of his theories to unsolved and often ignored problems in physics and biology, writes:

> [L]*iving matter has remained within the boundary of classical intuition so that the possibility of using the quantum theory in describing the behaviour and organization of the elementary components of living things has been overlooked by the mainstream of science.*[31]

Working in Milan, Italy, with Giuliano Preparata, DelGuidice has developed a new approach to understanding how matter can work together in a coherent way. This theory, called *super radiance*, describes a collective motion of matter coupled to an electromagnetic field using a quantum approach. In quantum theory, an object in its ground state is not at rest, but subject to internal fluctuations. The super radiance model postulates an interaction of the fluctuations of all the components (objects) within a so-called coherence domain which involves the electromagnetic field. DelGuidice suggests that in the future, this idea may be applied to provide a quantum-based framework for biology. From a sketch of his new approach, we can see that it deals not with how fields affect individual molecules, but with how fields help them work together as a whole.

The late Dr. Herbert Fröhlich, working at the University of Liverpool, has played a key role in the development of new physical approaches to the understanding of biological organization. Fröhlich has pioneered the concept of "coherent excitations" and how it applies to understanding how living systems work together as a whole. Fröhlich's mathematical theory describes how a system of molecules can be affected by energy from such sources as electromagnetic fields in such a way as to create order in all the molecules. Other scientists have explored Fröhlich's basic ideas both in theory and in experiments. There is emerging experimental evidence for the Fröhlich model,[32] despite a grave lack of research funds for such basic research and, for the most part, little interest among scientists.

Fröhlich's "coherent excitations" could be applied in important ways to biology. For example, one application of this idea is in understanding the interaction between enzymes, the protein workhorses of our cells, and the molecules with which they interact (called *substrates*). A selective long-range interaction between enzyme and substrate may arise from the theory of coherent excitations. This could help to explain the very effective chemical activity of enzymes. The basic idea of enzyme-substrate interaction is that the substrate fits neatly into a space in the enzyme, described as a "lock and key" interaction. The substrate is chemically altered by the influence of the enzyme — this is the enzyme's important job. One problem, though, has always been that it was hard to understand how the "key" found the "lock" in the first place, since biological molecules are thought to undergo random thermal motion. Fröhlich's model, which predicts that the enzyme and substrate attract each other by a long-range interaction, would explain how the key finds the lock.

Fröhlich discussed his theory with respect to the problem of cancer.[33] He suggested that understanding the control of cell growth is important in cancer research and that long-range interactions between cells must be involved. Further, he postulated that the control could be related to the excitation of specific vibrations in the organs or tissues involved. Could the successful development of Fröhlich's ideas mean that illnesses will be treated in the future by the application of specific electromagnetic frequencies?

This area of research is still in its infancy however, and with little support, monetary or otherwise, from the mainstream. The emergence of a mechanism for specific effects of low-energy fields on biological systems may indeed lie in this realm, but should not be expected in the near future.

Biological Circuits

Two men, both medical doctors as well as researchers, have separately suggested that their experiments demonstrate the existence of electric circuits other than the well-known nervous system. Dr. Björn Nordenström, a Swedish radiology professor, has hypothesized the existence of what he calls "biologically closed electric circuits," based on animal experiments and clinical research.[34] He describes pathways of conduction for various ions in the blood vessels and lymphatic system, which exist at both microscopic and macroscopic levels and form a complex network. In Nordenström's model these circuits are important for both structural and functional aspects of biological matter.

Biologically closed electric circuits are a flow of charges (current) which thereby generate magnetic fields. Nordenström feels that environmental electromagnetic fields can interact with the magnetic fields produced by the biologically closed electric circuits. Therefore, he concludes that environmental fields can influence the body. His ideas have attracted little attention, although his use of electricity as a treatment for cancer, based on his theory, seems to have generated some interest.

Another medical doctor, Dr. Robert Becker, has studied the electrical properties associated with tissue injury and regeneration, and as the result of his work postulates the existence of biological circuitry.[35] Based on research on a variety of animals, Becker describes a direct current (DC) analog system of electrical control. In his model, the DC currents, which are thought to be involved in the process of healing, are carried in perineural cells. These types of cells are found in close association with neurons in the brain and surround the nerve cells of the peripheral nervous system. Becker suggests that this second system regulates and controls the nerve-impulse system in the body and is a more primitive, but higher level of organismic organization. The existence of such a system of control may provide a means for an interaction of living things with weak energy fields. Again, little attention has been paid to this research.

CONCLUSION: THE DEBATE OF A NEW FRONTIER

Some insight into the controversy might be gained by highlighting the debate at a June 25, 1991 meeting of the Bioelectromagnetics Society, as reported by Dr. Beverly Rubik, Director of the Centre for Frontier Sciences at Temple University, Philadelphia.[36] This meeting addressed the question of ELF bioeffects. The invited speakers presented diverse opinions, as Rubik describes, ranging from those who are actively researching for mechanisms of interaction to those who are sceptical that effects even exist at all, except from very strong fields.

Dr. Arthur Pilla of Mt. Sinai Medical Centre, a researcher studying low-frequency field effects on bone repair, presented a model of field interaction at the level of the cell membrane involving cell communication. Dr. Dean Astumian, a scientist from the National Institute of Sciences and Technology, discussed a model of interaction that demonstrated a response in particular membrane proteins to weak electric fields. Rubik described a third lecture by Dr. Eberhard Neumann, a German scientist who also developed a model of the interaction of biological systems with weak fields.

In contrast to these active bioelectromagnetics researchers, a presentation by Dr. Robert Park, a physicist from the University of Maryland, suggested that weak fields cannot possibly produce biological effects. He came to this conclusion because of the thermal noise objection. He criticized the cyclotron resonance model from the same angle and indicated that effects showing frequency, intensity and temperature windows are not possible. Further, from his analysis of epidemiology he indicated his opinion that other factors were probably responsible for positive results and pointed out that power line fields represent only a small part of a typical daily field exposure. Park dismissed bioeffects as being against the laws of physics and epidemiological studies as being very weak.

The debate following Park's lecture was described by Rubik as "heated". Researchers, many of whom have been active in bioelectromagnetics for some time, dismissed his arguments as oversimplified. They pointed out some epidemiological surveys have examined confounding factors with no change in outcome. Further, they pointed out that organisms have evolved an exquisite sensitivity to the signals in their environment where sensory systems like the auditory system have evolved to overcome problems with noise. Ross Adey, who was also in attendance, compared Park's analysis to high-school physics, and described the various areas of modern physics not considered by Park. The final paragraph of Rubik's report of this meeting is insightful:

A final general discussion followed. Mechanisms ranging from magnetite microcrystals as field detectors in tissues to cyclotron resonance, were proposed. Clearly, there is little agreement on mechanisms for biological effects from low level ELF fields, as the debate from this session remains unresolved. On the other hand, as I have frequently observed in controversies from other frontier science areas, the arguments raised by the mainstream show that they are generally much less informed than those actively working in the field. Indeed, the history of biophysics has shown many aspects of physics that seem to have been confounded by the evolution of life. Life evolved specific mecha-

nisms to overcome what were once perceived as "physics blocks". If the thermal noise limit is indeed an issue, then it may be that life may have managed to evolve some mechanism to overcome it, a mechanism which, in my opinion, remains obscure to us at this time.[36]

CHAPTER 4 NOTES

1. Becker, R.O. and G. Selden (1985) *The Body Electric: Electromagnetism and the Foundation of Life.* New York: William Morrow and Company, 336.

2. An electrical device can produce an electric field when plugged into an outlet, even though the device is switched off. This depends on where the switch is placed relative to the live and neutral wires of the home's electrical wiring. A device called a demand switch can be used to disconnect a home's electrical wiring when no devices are in use, thereby eliminating electric fields for this period of time.

3. For further reading see: Anderson, L.E. (1991) "Biological Effects of Extremely Low-Frequency Electromagnetic Fields: *In Vivo* Studies." In Bierbaum, P.J., and J.M. Peters, eds. *Proceedings of the Scientific Workshop on the Health Effects of Electric and Magnetic Fields on Workers*, held by the National Institute of Occupational Safety and Health in Cincinnati. NIOSH Publication No. 91-111.

4. There are three different types of magnetism: paramagnetism, diamagnetism and ferromagnetism. In most atoms, the magnetic effects of the electrons, which are moving charges, will cancel each other out. This results in a non-magnetic ion or atom. In paramagnetism, however, the magnetic effects of the electrons do not cancel each other out. Aluminium, manganese, calcium, chromium and oxygen are some of the elements which are paramagnetic.

Diamagnetism was discovered in 1846 by Michael Faraday during an experiment in which he brought a sample of bismuth close to the pole of a strong magnet. He discovered that they repelled each other. He called this phenomenon diamagnetism. When an atom is placed in a magnetic field, one particular direction of electron rotation is preferred. This preferred rotation of the electron will result in the fields not cancelling each other out, giving rise to diamagnetism. Bismuth, lead, gold and zinc are examples of elements that are diamagnetic.

In ferromagnetism, a special type of interaction (exchange coupling) occurs between adjacent atoms that couple together their magnetic moments in a parallel fashion. Thus, in ferromagnetism, there is a high degree of magnetic alignment. This type of magnetism can occur in iron, copper and nickel, and alloys of these three elements.

5. The magnetic field strength, H, is another physical quantity that is used to describe magnetism. There is a close relationship between B and H, where one can be calculated from the other when the magnetic properties of the material in which the fields occur is known. The magnetic flux density (B) is measured in units of tesla or gauss, whereas the magnetic field strength (H) is measured in units of amperes per metre.

6. Maxwell's equations represent the most compact set of laws that encompass ordinary electromagnetism. Physicists often describe these equations as having a certain beauty, as they connect experiments in a wide area and are able to predict new outcomes. The scope of these equations ranges from the basic principles of motors to television and radio. Maxwell's four equations describe electric and magnetic fields, the electrical effect of a changing magnetic field, and symmetrically the magnetic effect of a changing electric field.

7. In an electromagnetic wave the electric (E) and magnetic (B) fields are perpendicular to each other. The direction in which the wave travels is in turn perpendicular to the plane of these two fields.

8. The formula $E = hf$ is the basic relationship between the energy (E) and the frequency (f) of the wave. The letter h represents Planck's constant. This is a fundamental constant equal to 6.626×10^{-34} Js. This formula was first suggested by Einstein in the early 1900s and helped him win a Nobel prize in 1921.

9. There are direct and indirect pathways for biological effects from ionizing radiation. A direct effect occurs when the target molecule/atom is directly altered in its chemical makeup by incoming radiation. Indirect effects occur when a biological molecule is damaged by another molecule that has itself been directly affected by the radiation. For example, radiation-produced free radicals can damage DNA by rupturing the sugar-phosphate bonds comprising the backbone of the DNA molecule.

10. Electric Power Research Institute (1990) *Electric and Magnetic Field Research*, 12.

11. Nair, M., G. Morgan and H.K. Florig (1989) "Biological Effects of Power Frequency Electric and Magnetic Fields: Background Paper." Washington: United States Congress, Office of Technology Assessment, Report No. OTA-BP-E-53.

12. A basic relation between electric field E and voltage V is V=Ed,

where d is a separation over which the voltage is measured. From this equation, E=V/d and from this it can be seen that if d is a very small number like the width of a cell membrane, E will be very large.

13. The reader is referred to the following: Persinger, M.A. (1974) *VLF and ELF Electromagnetic Fields Effects.* New York: Plenum Press. This book also contains a paper by R. Wever on cave experiments and circadian rhythms.

Adey, W.R. (1981) "Tissue Interactions with Non-Ionizing Electromagnetic Fields." *Physiological Reviews* 61:2.

14. Adey, W.R. (1990) "Joint Actions of Environmental Non-ionizing Electromagnetic Fields and Chemical Pollution in Cancer Promotion." *Environmental Health Perspectives* 86, 297-305.

15. Weaver, J. and R.D. Astumian (1990) "The Response of Living Cells to Very Weak Electric Fields: The Thermal Noise Limit." *Science* 247, 459-461.

16. Dr. J.L. Kirschvink, a professor of geobiology at the California Institute of Technology in Pasadena, discovered magnetite crystals in the human brain. *Frontier Perspectives* 3:1, Fall 1992, 39.

17. Adair, R.K. (1991) "Constraints on Biological Effects of Weak Extremely-Low-Frequency Electromagnetic Fields." *Physical Review A.* 43:2, 1039-1048.

Kirschvink, J.L. (1992) "Comment on 'Constraints on Biological Effects of Weak Extremely-Low-Frequency Electromagnetic Fields'." *Physical Review A.* 46:4, 2178-2184.

Adair, R.K. (1992) "Reply to 'Comment on "Constraints on Biological Effects of Weak Extremely-Low-Frequency Electromagnetic Fields"'." *Physical Review A.* 46:4, 2185-2187.

18. Electric Power Research Institute (1990) "The Cyclotron Resonance Hypothesis: An EMF Health Effects Resource Paper."

19. Liboff, A.R. (1985) "Cyclotron Resonance in Membrane Transport." In Chiaberera, A. Nicolini, C. and H.P. Schwan, eds. *Interactions Between Electromagnetic Fields and Cells.* New York: Plenum Press.

20. Thomas, J.R., J. Schrot and A.R. Liboff. (1986) "Low Intensity Magnetic Fields Alter Operant Behaviour in Rats." *Bioelectromagnetics 7*, 349-357.

21. Marino, A.A. (1988) "Environmental Electromagnetic Energy and Public Health." In Marino, A.A., ed. *Modern Bioelectricity.* Marcel Decker Inc.

22. "The British Columbia Utility Commission on ELF Health Effects." July 11, 1989, 21.

23. Wilson, B.W., E.K. Chess and L.E. Anderson (1986) "60 Hz Elec-

tric Field Effects on Pineal Melatonin Rhythms: Time Course for Onset and Recovery." *Bioelectromagnetics* 7, 239-242.

24. Bierbaum, P.J., and J.M. Peters, eds. (1991) *Proceedings of the Scientific Workshop on the Health Effects of Electric and Magnetic Fields on Workers*, held by the National Institute of Occupational Safety and Health in Cincinnati. NIOSH Publication No. 91-111.

25. Vena, J. *et al.* (1991) "Use of Electric Blankets and Risk of Postmenopausal Breast Cancer." *American Journal of Epidemiology* 134, 180-185. Cited in *Microwave News* (1991) 11:5, 3.

26. *Microwave News* (1990) 10:4, 9.

27. Adey, W.R. (1989) *Cell Membranes, Electromagnetic Fields and Intercellular Communications*. Springer Series in Brain Dynamics. Springer Verlag.

28. Some scientists have even commented on whether the assumption holds that biological systems should always be described by the laws of physics. For example, physicist Dr. Herbert Fröhlich's short essay "Can Biology Accommodate Laws Beyond Physics?" and "Some Epistemological Issues in Physics and Biology" by the biologist Dr. Robert Rosen, both address this question. These papers appear in Hiley, B.J. and D. Peat, eds. (1987) *Quantum Implications: Essays in Honour of David Bohm*. London: Routledge and Kegan Paul. Rosen, for example, discusses the implications of understanding complex biological systems in terms of simple sub-systems. Perhaps, he suggests "it is physics that has to be modified in order to deal with organic phenomena."

29. Smith, C.W. and S. Best (1989) *Electromagnetic Man: Health and Hazard in the Electrical Environment*. New York: St. Martin's Press.

Popp, F.A. *et al.* (1989) *Electromagnetic Bioinformation*. Munich: Urban and Schwarzenberg.

Fröhlich, H., ed. (1988) *Biological Coherence and Response to External Stimuli*. Berlin: Springer Verlag.

30. Adey, W.R. (1987) "Evidence for Tissue Interactions with Microwave and Other Non-Ionizing Electromagnetic Fields in Cancer Promotion." In *The Biophysics of Cancer*. Prague: Charles University.

Adey, W.R. (1990) "Joint Actions of Environmental Nonionizing Electromagnetic Fields and Chemical Pollution in Cancer Promotion." *Environmental Health Perspectives* 86, 297-305.

31. *Frontier Perspectives* (1990) 1:2.

32. Fröhlich, H., ed. (1988) *Biological Coherence and Response to External Stimuli*. Berlin: Springer Verlag.

33. Fröhlich, H. (1978) "Theoretical Physics and Biology." In Fröhlich, H., ed. (1988) *Biological Coherence and Response to External Stimuli*. Berlin: Springer Verlag.

34. Nordenström. B. (1991) "Bioelectrical Circuits in the Body." In *Frontier Perspectives* 2:2, 16.

35. Becker, R.O. (1990) *Cross Currents: The Promise of Electromagnetism, the Perils of Electropollution.* Los Angeles: Jeremy P. Tarcher Inc.

36. Rubik. B. (1991) "BEMS Symposium Explores Mechanisms for ELF Electromagnetic Bioeffects." *Frontier Perspectives* 2:2, 1.

FIVE

PUBLIC DIMENSIONS

There is a Faustian bargain inherent in our technological efforts. Each new technology brings both the power to direct the world around us for our selfish goals and the potential for our self-destruction. An acute realization of the extent of this bargain has manifested itself in the past few decades and we have collectively begun to come to grips with the impact of our technologies on planetary and personal health. The 1992 Earth Summit held in Rio de Janeiro demonstrated there is widespread agreement on the imminent danger to planetary health, even though the historic gathering proved to be weak on solutions.

There is a pattern to our technological development. We invent a new technology, certain of its great benefits. While we may be aware of some acute risks from the beginning, we cannot fully estimate the long-term consequences of this technology. Industry energetically promotes the benefits of the new technology, ignoring or downplaying the bad side. This initiates a consumer frenzy as the rush begins to be the first to possess the new and exciting technology. Even those affected by the negative impact have only a brief opportunity to lament the "price of progress" as the new technology becomes a basic necessity of life. Years later as the full impact becomes clearer it is too late to go back. A weak call is sometimes raised for more vigilance in evaluating new technologies — for us to control, rather than be controlled by, our discoveries. Yet a sense of technological determinism predominates: progress must come at all costs.

Electricity follows this pattern. It is too late to go back to a time where we didn't use it every day, and there is no question of doing so. Instead we have to learn to live with the new knowledge, some hundred years after the introduction of Thomas Alva Edison's system of electric power, that the electromagnetic fields created by our electrical networks seem to be harmful to our health. We have learned to live with all the other risks related to our use of electricity — shock hazards, coal mining, nuclear power . . . Ironically, the early debates over whose electrical system was better — Edison's DC system or George Westinghouse's AC system — focused on which was safer for the public. The Westinghouse AC approach won the day even though it was later shown to indeed be more hazardous (in terms of shock), as his bitter rival Edison had always claimed. And a further irony is that there is once again discussion of whether DC is safer than AC electricity, but this time in terms of the fields they produce.

There are several stages in the process of learning to live with the risks of new technologies. Risks related to many illnesses like cancer only become apparent after many years or even decades. The first stage is for scientific research to define and quantify these often subtle risks and to understand how these risks come about. The beginning then is the discovery of the side-effects of technology, and these discoveries are never greeted with the same enthusiasm as the new technologies themselves were. And when the discoveries of risks are made directly by the people most affected, there has historically been even less acceptance (until a subsequent "rediscovery" or confirmation by science).

In Chapter 3, we described some of the research that is being done on the effects of electromagnetic fields on living organisms. One major feature of this research, which we have tried to emphasize, is its controversial nature within the scientific community itself. One of the enduring myths about science is the idea that there are cold, hard facts which reveal easily demonstrable truths. However, the scientific process is more like a jigsaw puzzle, with each new study adding one more piece to the picture. Occasionally new observations which don't fit neatly into the existing picture come along, forcing us to overturn the whole game and begin again.

Interpretation is as much a part of science as the data it's based on. Working from the same experimental results, scientists can draw a wide range of conclusions. How the jigsaw is constructed into a comprehensible and meaningful landscape depends on other factors besides the actual data. There are many influences on the scientific research that represents this first stage of learning to live with technologies. In the case of electromagnetic fields from electrical and electromagnetic technologies, the observation that these weak fields can affect living organisms at all challenges fundamental ideas in science. Also, there are basic questions about the extent to which research on risks from technologies is even carried out and if so, who should pay for it. Further questions can be raised about the validity of the results of research carried out by the industries involved: too often the fox gets to guard the chickens. Part of the historical pattern has been for society to deal with problems long after industries have comfortably retired with their profits. In any case, our successful economic future is thought to be tied to our successful development of new technologies, and this, whether fact or fiction, means that little effort remains to focus on the social, ecological and health impact of technologies past, present, and future.

The public plays a role in this scientific process. As issues enter the public domain and become political and legal matters, public concern helps make available more funding for research. With increased funding, encouragement is provided for scientists who want to undertake the kind of research required. Public reaction plays an important role in determining whether a particular question gets attention. Certainly many people are starting to show concern about the effects of our continual contact with electromagnetic fields in our homes and workplaces, from power lines, electric blankets, household wiring and our ever-increasing use of electromagnetic technology.

The second part of the process of learning to live with the risks from technologies follows naturally from the first, but to some extent occurs simultaneously. In the first stage, the discovery of risks is elaborated on to the extent where we can determine exactly what the risks are in all different situations. The second stage involves the engineering problem of studying the technology, determining how it can be changed to lower risks, and how much these changes will cost. In the case of electromagnetic fields and health, scientists are beginning to understand more about how fields affect living organisms, and the risks of contact with the fields in our environment. While there is more to learn about these questions, engineers have begun to study how environmental fields can be reduced and how much these changes cost. Since power lines have been the main focus, most of the work has dealt with determining risks from power line fields, learning more about ways to reduce fields and to study the costs involved.

A specific example from electromagnetic field risks will help to demonstrate these first stages. The Feychting-Ahlbom study of power line fields and cancer (see Chapter 3) showed a link between magnetic fields and childhood leukemia. It was a powerful study because it found a dose-response relationship — exposure to stronger magnetic fields meant higher risks. A dose-response relationship means an association between magnetic fields and childhood cancer can be more confidently made, and the risks from different fields can be more precisely determined. The Feychting-Ahlbom study prompted Jaak Nou, the Director of Electrical Safety for the Swedish National Board for Industrial and Technological Development, to comment that a field-cancer link is 80 per cent certain and that his board must take action now and not wait until the 100 per cent level is achieved.[1] Nou was quoted in the *New Scientist* saying that because of the Feychting-Ahlbom study, he will proceed on the assumption that there is a link between power line magnetic fields and childhood leukemia. In the first stage of the risk process, Nou noted that in the Swedish population as a whole, 3.5 new cases of childhood leukemia could be expected each year and as an example of the second stage, that he will make a careful study of the costs of reducing exposures in a report to the government.

The third stage is where the real decisions are made about what to do about a technological risk problem — it is an area called risk analysis and management, and there are experts who specialize in this area. Risk management is where all the politics surrounding the interaction of industry, government and the public take place. Here the costs and benefits of technologies are brought to the table and decisions are made about whether to do anything about risks and if so, how much to spend. The precise data on risk and the costs of risk reduction are combined with human and social values to make real decisions affecting our lives. Clearly this is an area where the public not only deserves to be involved but should demand to be involved.

But two factors have worked against such involvement. Many members of the public find it easy to enjoy technologies and ignore the ecological and personal risks, and in deferring to the "price of progress", leave questions of risks to the experts. Also, many experts in risk management have felt that the public is not well enough informed about basic questions of risk to warrant inclusion in the decisions. These experts have based these conclusions on their own studies and often have a close connection to industry. There is an obvious need for public involvement in risk management decisions and fortunately there is a movement in risk management towards this end. Before we explore examples of how the electromagnetic fields and health issue has entered the public domain, we can highlight the need for public involvement in risk management decisions by quoting Dr. M. Granger Morgan, head of the Department of Engineering and Public Policy at Carnegie Mellon University and a researcher long involved in risk analysis and management. Morgan represents this positive and long overdue trend for a recognition of the importance of public involvement in deciding how we "manage" the technologies around us.

My experience and that of my colleagues indicate that the public can be very sensible about risk when companies, regulators and other institutions give it the opportunity. Laypeople have different, broader definitions of risk, which in important respects can be more rational than the narrow ones used by experts. Furthermore, risk management is, fundamentally, a question of values. In a democratic society, there is no acceptable way to make these choices without involving the citizens who will be affected by them.[2]

THE NEW YORK STATE POWER LINES PROJECT

In 1973, the New York State Public Service Commission received applications from two private sector corporations for the construction of a pair of 765 kV high-voltage transmission lines. The proposed power lines were larger than the ones in use at that time — up to 345 kV lines were then in use in New York State — and public interest over the possibility of health effects from the new lines prompted public hearings.[3] A number of scientists were involved in these hearings, during which scientific research regarding the effects of low-level power-frequency electric and magnetic fields on biological systems was scrutinized by numerous lawyers and consultant scientists.

Five years later, in 1978, the commission finally ruled that the 765 kV lines could be built, provided that they would be surrounded by a 350-foot right-of-way within which homes could not be built. This size of the right-of-way was determined by the fact that the electric field at the edge of such a corridor would be about the same strength as the electric field at the edge of a 345 kV right-of-way. The commissioners felt that the public was prepared to accept a level of exposure comparable to that created by lines already in existence at that time. The commission considered only electric fields; magnetic fields created by the power line were not considered.

The most significant outcome of the hearings was the panel's recommendation that the utility fund a research program to help determine possible human health risks from overhead power transmission lines. This led to the establishment in 1980 of the New York State Power Lines Project. Administered by the New York State Department of Health under the direction of Dr. David O. Carpenter, the Project was given a $5 million budget.

A panel of scientists was selected from a wide range of disciplines. This panel was to review the current knowledge of health effects from power line frequencies and identify the most important research areas. After reviewing almost 200 proposals from researchers, the panel awarded sixteen research contracts. The research projects included studies of cells, behavioural effects, circadian rhythms, and childhood leukemia.

Of the resulting studies, one epidemiological survey of adult cancer in Seattle found no association between electromagnetic fields and adult cancers, and no effects from electromagnetic fields were found on reproduction, growth and development. Studies investigating genetic or chromosomal damage in cells also failed to observe any effects.

However, other studies did observe effects. Small effects on the brain chemistry of monkeys were found. Additionally, effects from fields were observed on biological rhythms, the response of rats to pain, and the learning ability of rats.[3] Dr. David Savitz's study of the relationship between power line fields and childhood leukemia captured the most attention. Savitz found that children living near high-current power lines had 2.1 times the incidence of leukemia as children who did not live near these lines. "What the study does do is significantly strengthen the hypothesis that electromagnetic fields cause cancer," declared Carpenter, the man who had been chosen to head the Power Lines Project, although he cautioned, "Far more research must be done before we have any conclusive proof."[4]

Among the panel's recommendations, contained in its final report issued in 1987, was the suggestion that a major research effort be launched on the delivery of power with reduced magnetic field exposure. The final report pointed to avenues of research on electromagnetic field bioeffects that should be explored, and recommended that research should be administered by a federal agency which is "clearly independent of partisan influence."[3]

THE POWER LINE CONTROVERSY
ON VANCOUVER ISLAND

In the mid 1980s British Columbia Hydro proposed to build a 230 kV transmission line on Vancouver Island. The regulatory review process for the new line began in 1987, with little public attention. Then, in the spring of 1988, two homeowners along the proposed right-of-way publicly voiced their objections to the proposal. After examining information provided by BC Hydro, one of the residents said he was unwilling to accept any health risks that might be associated with the new line. A second resident along the right-of-way began to campaign publicly about the potential dangers from the proposed line. As a result, the provincial regulatory agency considering BC Hydro's proposal, the British Columbia Utilities Commission, received further complaints.

At this point, BC Hydro released information from its own files on the public health aspects of the proposal, and allowed certain personnel to become publicly involved in the debate so that homeowners could decide for themselves whether a possible health hazard existed. BC Hydro even offered to buy the properties of any residents whose misgivings over the power line were not put to rest by the information made available to them. However, this remarkable move on the part of the utility backfired, as many residents took this as an admission of adverse health consequences of living near a power line. Of 144 property owners receiving such a purchase offer, 66 accepted, and another 140 who were not included in the buy-out offer responded as well.

In 1989, in response to all this, the Utilities Commission launched a public inquiry into the new line; construction on the line was stopped until after the public hearings, which began in July 1989.[5] Between 125 and 180 people attended the hearings, and as noted in the commission's final report, the community showed deep concern over the low-frequency field health issue. The inquiry featured testimony by Dr. Andrew Marino, who was brought in on behalf of a group of concerned residents,[6] as well as two consultant scientists hired by BC Hydro. The commission also hired an independent epidemiologist to advise them in their deliberations.

BC Hydro took the position that electromagnetic field bioeffects science was quite new and showed no consistent pattern of results, and that no definitive conclusions could be drawn until much more research had been carried out. The consultants retained by BC Hydro presented a similarly conservative point of view. One of these consultants disputed the New York State Power Lines Project report's conclusion that the Savitz study of childhood leukemia indicated a strong possibility of a connection between low-frequency magnetic fields and childhood cancer.[5] The conclusions of the Wertheimer and Leeper childhood leukemia study were also questioned. In the opinion of the BC Hydro consultants, the new power line "posed no risk to human health."[5]

Andrew Marino told the commission that the new power line presented a health risk in the context of his stressor hypothesis. He said absolute proof of causality may be virtually impossible, but evidence pointed strongly to the fact that magnetic fields were risk factors for cancer. Marino also testified that the health impact of chronic field exposure should be considered with respect to all the other risk factors present in the environment. He felt that judgments should be based on a consideration of all the possible risk factors associated with human disease, and that an excessive reaction on the part of the public to electromagnetic fields was not necessary.[5]

One of the consultants hired by BC Hydro challenged Marino's stressor hypothesis. There is no evidence that electric or magnetic fields were stressors, he stated; in order to be considered a chronic stressor, a factor must first be demonstrated to be an acute stressor. In his view, there are no differences between acute and chronic stressors — the acute stressor becomes a chronic one as the exposure duration is lengthened.

The inquiry's final report stressed that the electromagnetic field and health issue must be seen in the light of overall human exposure to low-frequency electromagnetic fields, including the use of appliances. Electric blankets and heated waterbeds were specifically referred to. "[T]here is cause for concern within the scientific literature about the biological effects on humans of electromagnetic radiation," the report stated. "There is, however, insufficient evidence to support a presumption of an actual health risk."[5]

The commission's report also cited a lack of coordination in Canadian electromagnetic field health research. About $100 million had been spent worldwide on studies without conclusive results, the report said; establishing standards of acceptable exposure for power line fields would either provoke unwarranted alarm or create a false sense of security.

The final report rejected calls to underground the new line in order to reduce low-frequency fields on the grounds that this could increase construction costs up to twenty times, an expense which the commission felt was not justified by the evidence it had heard. Proposals to reroute the line away from population centres were also rejected. This line was to serve a new newsprint mill, and the commission viewed the keeping of the delivery schedule for the power as an important factor in their decision.

The final recommendations pointed to the emotional strain on those members of the public involved. Inquiry Chairman John G. McIntyre expressed his view that the "moderate" comments of Savitz, echoed at times by Marino, that there is no need for public alarm, were of limited consolation to individuals who wanted categorical assurances of safety. The commission suggested that if children were discouraged from extended periods of play within a power line right-of-way, this would be consistent with the "prudent avoidance" policy recommended in a 1989 US Congressional Office of Technology Assessment report ("prudent avoidance" is discussed in Chapter 6). The inquiry report stressed the fact that magnetic fields decrease rapidly with distance, and exposures can be minimized simply by not getting too close to the source of these fields.

McIntyre's report broadened the issue over the fields from the new line. He pointed out that high-voltage power line fields are not substantially different from the background magnetic fields produced by household wiring and appliances. In some cases, neighbourhood distribution lines can create significant magnetic fields. McIntyre castigated the utility for its buy-out scheme, citing among other things its impact in heightening concern rather than its intended effect of amelioration. BC Hydro's inconsistency in deciding which homes were to be presented with a purchase offer was criticized. It was recommended that the utility fund research to complement such work elsewhere and develop public awareness programs.

THE U.S. ENVIRONMENTAL PROTECTION AGENCY REPORT

In its effort to respond to public safety questions surrounding environmental low-frequency electromagnetic fields, the United States Environmental Protection Agency (EPA) reviewed and evaluated the available scientific literature for several years and formulated a draft report, entitled "An Evaluation of the Potential Carcinogenicity of Electromagnetic Fields," which was scheduled for release in the spring of 1990. The draft version of this report concluded there was a significant link between low-frequency magnetic field exposure and cancer, enough in fact, to warrant classification of ELF fields as "probable human carcinogens." Such a categorization placed these fields with PCBs and formaldehyde in the EPA's classification scheme for cancer-causing agents.

This classification was edited out of the final version of the report by the EPA's Director of Health and Environmental Assessment, Dr. William Farland. A copy of the draft report was leaked to the media, and Farland was forced to defend the deletion. He did so on the basis of the fact that the exact mechanism of interaction between electromagnetic fields and biological systems was not known, and in the absence of a clear relationship between exposure and response, such a classification was inappropriate. The final report did include the following statement:

In conclusion, several studies showing leukaemia, lymphoma, and cancer of the nervous system in children exposed to magnetic fields from residential 60Hz electrical distribution systems supported by similar findings in adults in several occupational studies also involving electrical power frequency exposures, show a consistent pattern of response that suggests a causal link.[7]

Even before its release, the report had attracted a lot of attention. The draft report was reviewed by the EPA's Science Advisory Board. The president's science advisor became involved, with another review set up by the committee on Inter-agency Radiation Research and Policy Coordination, an offshoot of the White House Office of Science and Technology Policy. Additionally, seven other federal agencies were asked to review the report.[8] Opinions of the report were divided.

The National Cancer Institute and Department of Defence both strongly criticized the EPA draft report. "In our judgement the conclusions presented remain scientifically unsound and unnecessarily alarming," declared the National Cancer Institute, while the Department of Defence said flatly that "This report should not be published."

However, other agencies responded more positively to the EPA report, including the Food and Drug Administration and the National Institute of Standards and Technology. The FDA concluded that "This is a well-researched document which presents a reasonable and balanced examination of the evidence available to date," while the reviewer for the National Institute of Standards and Technology commented, "I see no serious problem with issuing the book as it stands." Other reviewers included the Department of Energy, Department of Transportation and Occupational Safety and Health Administration.[8]

The Science Advisory Board established a new committee, the Non-ionizing Electric and Magnetic Field Subcommittee, to review the EPA report.[9] It held three public hearings to elicit input for its evaluation. The first, held early in 1991 in Washington, D.C., attracted more than 200 persons for presentations and opportunities to debate the EPA's conclusions with subcommittee members. Subsequent meetings were held in San Antonio, Texas and back in Washington, where additional presentations were heard and preliminary drafts on physics, biology and epidemiology were received.

The subcommittee's review of the EPA report cited "serious deficiencies" in the EPA's work, and said the report should be completely rewritten. It concluded that there was still a limited understanding of how electromagnetic fields of this type could affect living things, and a lack of a well-defined relationship between the exposure and biological response. As a result of these deficiencies, the subcommittee did not feel that a cause and effect relationship could be inferred with respect to magnetic fields and cancer. These deficiencies made epidemiological associations, based on magnetic field surrogates (like wire coding and job classification), fall short of demonstrating a proven link between magnetic fields and cancer. It also cited the opinion that many steps in the process of electromagnetic field biointeraction are unknown, and that the kinds of biological effects now observed cannot be used as evidence of a deleterious effect on human health, especially cancer.

The subcommittee acknowledged that cellular and animal experiments do indeed demonstrate non-thermal biological effects from ELF fields, as well as from unmodulated and ELF-modulated radio frequencies. But though some hypotheses do exist for relating these effects to adverse health consequences, the subcommittee reiterated its concern over the poor understanding of all the steps in this process. Thus, it concluded that low-frequency electromagnetic fields should not be classified using the EPA scheme for carcinogens and that there was insufficient information to set safety guidelines.

Two recommendations ended the subcommittee assessment. The subcommittee was "unanimous in its belief that the question of electric and magnetic field effects on biological systems is important and exceptionally challenging" and felt that the EPA should completely rewrite the report for review by the Science Advisory Board.[9] A second recommendation stated that the EPA should carry out more work on radio wave and microwave radiation, a question that has received attention since the EPA was established in the early 1970s. The subcommittee described these fields as presenting "long known and well understood hazards against which users and the general public must be warned and protected."[9] Their recommendation also noted the fact that the whole issue of low-frequency magnetic and electric fields evolved from continued concern about the hazards of radio/microwave radiation. They stated that the EPA report is misleading in its implication that power line-frequency carcinogenicity is the major health issue related to non-ionizing fields. The subcommittee's opinion on this matter was that the public had been presented a distorted picture, since the issue of low-frequency fields is really part of the larger context of non-ionizing fields of all kinds.[10]

LEGAL ISSUES

> *Utilities across the country are feeling the heat. Since the mid 1980's, power companies have been involved in more than 100 lawsuits involving possible health hazards from transmission lines, especially those near schools. The patchwork of lawsuits, public hearings and local government rulings is having a direct impact.*[11]

— from *Transmission and Distribution,* a trade magazine for electrical utility managers

Electromagnetic Fields in the Courtroom

❖ In June 1990, a mother whose teenage daughter died of leukemia in 1987 filed a suit alleging that exposure to electromagnetic fields from power lines and a substation caused the girl's illness.[12]

❖ A Texas utility was sued in 1987 by a family alleging that the brain tumour of their 26-year-old son was caused by a high-voltage transmission line.[12]

❖ A lawsuit in Seattle, Washington, by Robert Strom, a former Boeing worker, asserted his leukemia was the result of his exposure to pulsed electromagnetic fields in his workplace. Among the many experts listed to testify were Dr. Robert Becker, Dr. David Savitz and Dr. Abraham Liboff. This case was settled out of court with Mr. Strom receiving $500,000 from Boeing.[12]

❖ On July 15, 1991, a Fulton County, Georgia jury decided to award a settlement to a couple in the amount of over four times that initially paid by the utility for land used for a transmission line right-of-way. The couple argued that the utility should recompense them for land extending past the right-of-way where low-frequency fields were above background levels.[8]

❖ A 1991 article in *Microwave News* reported that the number of police officers with legal claims suggesting that their cancers were related to the use of traffic speed radar devices had risen to eight.[8] For example, several Connecticut police officers had filed claims for workers' compensation, and a Wisconsin officer's widow had filed suit against the radar manufacturer.

❖ In January 1993, a Florida man launched a lawsuit against NEC America, the manufacturer of his cellular telephone. His suit alleged that his wife's death from brain cancer was related to her use of the cellular phone, which exposes the user to low levels of high-frequency electromagnetic energy.

Opinions on Lawsuits

Arthur Bryant, a lawyer involved in the electromagnetic field issue, has pointed out three trends which he sees developing.[11] His comments were reported in a June 1991 issue of *Transmission and Distribution*. Firstly, Bryant suggested that the scientific evidence for adverse health effects from electromagnetic energy was growing, with the number of epidemiological studies reaching "significant double digits." Secondly, he observed that public awareness and activism was gaining strength. Finally, he noted, the amount of litigation was growing.

Bryant outlined the different kinds of cases that are being brought before the courts. For example, cases dealing with the construction of new power lines show that property owners whose land is to be used for a new line may be concerned with health risks and the devaluation of their property.

A similar case discussed by Bryant involved a conflict between a school district and the local utility. Houston Lighting Power (Texas) built a power line over school property which ran within 100 meters of three schools. The line ran less than 50 meters from one of these schools. The school district was concerned about possible health effects, and when the company did not address their concerns satisfactorily, the district sued Houston Lighting Power. A jury decided in the school district's favour, awarding $104,000 compensation to the school district for the loss of property plus $25 million in punitive damages, and ordered Houston Lighting Power to move the power line. In its verdict, the jury sharply criticized the utility, suggesting it had acted indifferently and recklessly in failing to take the school district's concerns into consideration before it went ahead with the power line construction. (In a subsequent appeal, the order to move the line and the award for loss of property were upheld, but the large award for punitive damages was reversed on a legal technicality.)

Another legal opinion featured in the same issue of *Transmission and Distribution* was expressed by Thomas Watson, a senior partner in a law firm which has represented a number of plaintiffs in lawsuits against electrical utilities. Watson predicted that utilities would increasingly face legal challenges when they propose new power lines and try to acquire the land for right-of-ways. Watson felt that utilities may have to grapple with moratoriums on new power lines enacted by local authorities. He noted that legal actions may be undertaken based on trespass, since fields extend past the right-of-way, but that these probably will not win. Duty-to-warn and misrepresentation claims were also mentioned by Watson in the context of determining a utility's responsibility to inform the public of the electromagnetic field and health issue.

THE QUESTION OF MITIGATION

With growing public awareness of and concern over environmental electromagnetic fields, the question of electric and magnetic field mitigation continues to be raised. Power utilities have begun to investigate techniques and designs to reduce fields from power lines. Most of the emphasis is now on reducing magnetic fields, which are more difficult to shield than low-frequency electric fields.

Computer displays that incorporate shielding and cancellation techniques are increasingly available. Electric blanket manufacturers including Fieldcrest and Northern Electric (Sunbeam) have designed low-field models. A Massachusetts company, Safe Technologies Corporation, which specializes in low-radiation computer monitors, also sells an alarm clock that has a reduced level of low-frequency magnetic fields. An increasing demand for field reduction in consumer products should mean that more examples of this kind will be seen in the marketplace in the future.

The reduction of low-frequency fields in the workplace has only begun to be addressed. Most of the interest to date has been in assessing the actual levels of exposure. The 1991 National Institute of Occupational Safety and Health (NIOSH) conference on low-frequency fields in the workplace defined an agenda for future field reduction research.

Until now, only the thermal effects of higher frequencies such as radio and microwaves in the workplace have been considered. But with allegations that a number of police officers' cancers were related to the use of traffic speed radar units, which involve exposures to microwave intensities well below those required for heating, several police departments in the United States have been interested in reducing the microwave exposure of officers using these radar units. Exposure reduction could be accomplished both by using units with low microwave emissions as well as by positioning the unit so that the officer receives the smallest exposure possible.

Research on the non-thermal effects of non-ionizing electromagnetism is continuing. However, the establishment of precise risk evaluation and safety standards based on such an evaluation may still be many years away. The impetus for field mitigation then must be driven by other factors. Public interest may produce more consumer devices with reduced magnetic fields. The policy of "prudent avoidance" and the idea of "as low as reasonably achievable" (ALARA) will undoubtedly be major considerations for the short term. The major focus on mitigation has been low-frequency (ELF) fields, especially the magnetic fields from power lines.

Power Line Field Reduction

There are several major components of an electric power system. The first stage is called *generation*; this is where the electric power is produced, whether by hydroelectric, oil-fired, nuclear or other means. The electrical energy must be moved from the site of production to the cities and towns where it is needed. This is accomplished by the *transmission* system. It is more efficient to transmit power at high voltages; transmission lines use high voltages and can be identified by their large, often metal pylons. Once the electrical energy reaches a town or city, it enters the *distribution* system. The distribution system operates at a lower voltage, so the transmission line voltage is "stepped down" in a distribution substation. Distribution lines deliver power directly to the consumers. The distribution line voltage is again lowered to the 110/220 volts required in our homes using a transformer, typically a can-shaped unit mounted on a utility pole. Every part of the electrical power system produces electric and magnetic fields.

An example of one utility's response to electric and magnetic field reduction is provided by the construction of a new power line in Oregon in the early 1990s.[13] In order to respond to an increased demand for electricity in southern Oregon and northern California, PacifiCorp designed a 500 kV transmission line extending over 100 miles from Eugene to Medford. The line was to be completed by September 1993. After the construction permit for this line was issued, expressions of public concern forced the Oregon Department of Energy to instruct PacifiCorp to look into ways of reducing electromagnetic fields. In order to address "environmental and public concerns," the line's design incorporated features for reducing electric and magnetic fields. Pacifi-

Corp used a new line design, known as delta phase configuration, instead of a more common horizontal configuration (see Figure 7). Delta phase configuration lines reduced magnetic fields at the edge of the right-of-way by 45 per cent, and this was accomplished with a 1.5 per cent increase in construction costs.

Another example of the increasing emphasis on power line field reduction is the Electric Transmission Research Needs Task Force, created in 1990 by Washington's state legislature to study ways of reducing human electric and magnetic field exposure from electric power distribution systems. The final report of the Task Force represents an excellent source of information on field reduction knowledge and research.[14] It noted that low-frequency field exposures can be reduced either by engineering techniques — cancellation and shielding — discussed in the last chapter, or by increasing the distance between members of the public and field sources.

Regulations and policies encouraging exposure reduction have been adopted at state and local levels. Several states have guidelines for allowable fields at the edge of transmission line right-of-ways. Some state utility commissions have invoked "prudent avoidance" and "as low as reasonably achievable" as part of their strategies. For example, the Colorado Public Utilities Commission ordered its electric utilities to practice prudent avoidance by avoiding further exposures to fields where practical, and in New Jersey, utilities are required to demonstrate to the Department of Environmental Protection that field levels are as low as reasonably achievable.

There are several examples of city and county governments, and school districts attempting to address this issue. Lincolnwood, a Chicago suburb, has asked the local utility to limit magnetic fields to 1.5 mG and has placed a moratorium on the construction of new transmission lines in the meantime. The utility is challenging such directions. Several school districts have adopted measures addressing the concerns of parents. In three states, exposure levels for school yards have been proposed. In Montecito, California, some areas of an elementary

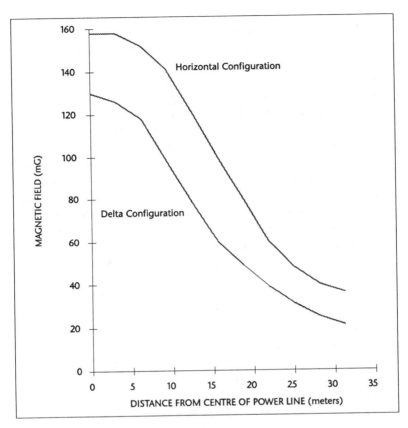

FIGURE 7

Magnetic fields near two types of transmission lines. The delta configuration has lower magnetic fields and has been used to help reduce environmental fields. *Adapted from:* Ferris, H.C. and K.D. Simpson, *Transmission and Distribution*, June 1991.

school were roped off after field measurements revealed higher-than-average readings.

One electric utility, Delmarva Power which serves parts of Delaware, Maryland and Virginia, has created self-imposed guidelines for the fields at the edge of transmission line right-of-ways. Other utilities provide information to the public on home field management and are looking at other means of reducing exposures. Seattle City Light, British Columbia Hydro, and Pacific Power and Light are mentioned in the Washington State Task Force report as having taken steps to reduce public exposures by rede-signing or expanding right-of-ways.

Serious study of electric and magnetic field exposure reduction techniques is underway as utilities, appliance manufacturers and other organizations respond to the discovery of a relationship between electromagnetic fields and health — the first stage in the process of living with technological risk. Knowledge of reduction techniques, the second stage, is required to provide the solutions determined by the third stage — risk management. A leading player in power line field exposure mitigation research is the Electric Power Research Institute (EPRI), which has spent more than $1 million researching ways of reducing magnetic field exposures from a range of sources.[14] EPRI is studying new designs for power lines that would result in reduced fields, as well as ways of reducing fields from existing lines. They have constructed a model residential neighbourhood to study magnetic field reduction, complete with a test house used to evaluate indoor magnetic fields. The role that grounding systems play in domestic magnetic fields is one aspect of this research effort. Another EPRI project is a U.S.-wide measurement survey designed to evaluate magnetic fields in homes.

In other EPRI-sponsored research, new remote-control equipment is being tested for use by utility workers. These devices will allow a worker to repair overhead transmission lines from the ground. Magnetic shielding is being studied for use in reducing magnetic field exposure of workers in cases where significant fields are encountered.

Research in New York State includes a study of the relationship between domestic magnetic fields and grounding in homes, as well as ways to help reduce residential exposures. In Florida, a task force is investigating field reduction for transmission lines. In California, a report before the legislature suggested that the state should address field reduction from power lines, household wiring and appliances since it is not clear which features of environmental fields may be of greatest importance in determining health consequences, or which field sources are most significant. In Sweden, the State Power Board is studying new transmission line designs to achieve significant field reductions. Other methods of cancelling fields from such lines are also being investigated.

The Washington State Task Force on Power Line Field Reduction

Highlights of the Washington State Task Force's report[14] on electric and magnetic field reduction will shed some light on the technical questions surrounding the reduction of power line fields. This Task Force did not address domestic field reduction. It did, however, point out that unbalanced ground return currents may be a major source of low-frequency magnetic fields in the home.

❖ The Task Force noted that in the past, electric and magnetic fields have not been a consideration when deciding the size of right-of-ways, although a wider right-of- way does mean weaker fields at the edge.

❖ Magnetic fields from power lines are related to the use of electricity by the public and industry and therefore show daily and seasonal variations. For example, measurements at a particular location in your home may be 0.8 mG in the early morning, and 1.1 mG around supper time.

❖ Many people incorrectly assume that undergrounding power lines will eliminate the fields: magnetic fields are not shielded by burial. However, the conductors in an undergrounded line can be brought closer together because they are insulated, so "cancellation" — orienting conductors in such a way that their fields cancel each other out

— reduces fields. Some partial shielding may occur if steel pipes are used, as in the case of fluid-insulated transmission cables.

❖ The degree of balance in a power line (in a balanced line the conductors carry equal and opposite currents[15]) is an important factor in determining the fields produced by the line. Moving the conductors closer together can help reduce fields, but balancing the lines achieves greater reduction. Transmission lines are generally more balanced than distribution lines. This is because distribution lines deliver power directly to homes and industries where the demand from the users of the electricity is constantly changing.

❖ Different designs of high-voltage transmission lines have a wide variation in the magnetic fields they produce (see Figure 8). The greatest field reductions for transmission lines are achieved by undergrounding in fluid-filled steel pipes. This eliminates electric fields and can reduce magnetic fields from the 29.7 mG of a standard design to 0.2 mG (for the line parameters used in the Washington State Task Force's evaluation) measured at 40 feet from the centre line. Directly above (or below) the lines, fields were 59.6 mG and 4.9 mG for standard and underground lines respectively. This reduction was found to be due to better cancellation, and not shielding. Unfortunately, this type of undergrounding can cost over seven times as much as a standard configuration.

❖ New types of overhead transmission lines could achieve

FIGURE 8 (Facing Page)
Comparison of cost and electromagnetic fields for three different transmission line designs. Costs are in U.S. dollars. Letters A, B and C in the design pictures represent the positions of the conductors. Adapted from: *Electric and Magnetic Field Reduction: Research Needs — A Report to the Washington State Legislature by the Electric Transmission Research Needs Task Force*, January 15, 1992.

Description	Picture of Design	Cost/Km in 1000s	Magnetic Field (mG)		Electric Field (kV/m)	
			under	*60 m*	*under*	*60 m*
1. Horizontal configuration - 230 kV - 300 amps - 125 MW		140-160	59.6	1.6	2.6	0.04
2. Delta configuration - 230 kV - 300 amps - 125 MW		135-155	28.9	0.5	1.6	0.03
3. Underground fluid-filled steel pipe - Buried 1.52 m underground		925-1250	4.9	0.01	0	0

reductions in the magnetic field from 4 to 16 times over standard designs. Such designs can cost 50 per cent more. Delta-type configurations for overhead lines can reduce fields by two to three times and are comparable in cost to standard designs. The most common design for transmission lines, the flat, horizontal configuration, results in the highest electric and magnetic fields.

❖ Burial of distribution lines, those lower-voltage lines that deliver power to consumers, does not result in the greatest reduction in magnetic fields. Several types of overhead designs for distribution lines create smaller magnetic fields than undergrounding. This is an interesting contrast to transmission lines.

Reducing Fields in the Workplace

The National Institute for Occupational Safety and Health has addressed research needs for measuring worker exposures to low-frequency magnetic and electric fields and for reducing workplace exposures.[16] At a 1991 NIOSH conference on Workplace Electric and Magnetic Fields the following recommendations were presented by a panel of scientists and engineers actively working in this area.

❖ Better methods for measuring exposures need to be developed.

❖ Sources of low-frequency fields in the workplace need to be identified and characterized.

❖ Changes in the electrical code relating to wiring practices designed to reduce electromagnetic field exposures need to be investigated.

❖ Further research is needed on work practices and field cancellation techniques for reducing workplace fields.

❖ More effective shielding materials and personal protective equipment need to be developed.

❖ Training programs to encourage field reduction need to

be developed. For example, future electrical engineers, trained in field reduction, could design low-field equipment, and workers, taught about electromagnetic field sources, would understand ways to reduce exposures.

STANDARDS AND GUIDELINES

It is often stated that there is "cause for concern" over environmental electromagnetic fields. Thus, the need for standards and guidelines has been raised. Yet the lack of scientific consensus and the many outstanding problems prevent a clear assessment of risks for given levels and types of exposures. Even scientists who feel that the present data demonstrate that a health hazard exists from exposure to non-ionizing energy at non-thermal intensities, often do not encourage standards and guidelines at this stage. Preliminary guidelines may create a false sense of security given the many outstanding questions. However, the public interest in preliminary guidelines and approaches for some level of public protection has meant that in several countries and states this issue has begun to be addressed.

Before we consider how the controversy over weak fields is being addressed, let us first look at protection efforts aimed at heating levels of radio and microwave fields. As we shall see, despite the fact that effects from these strong high-frequency fields are considered well established, the creation of safety standards is really a complex and political matter.

Thermal Effects Protection

In the 1950s, concern about human exposure to microwaves and radio waves resulted in the development of a set of standards governing exposure levels. In those days, it was thought that the only danger was from the heating of tissue, so safety standards were based on that. The earliest limits presented a single level of "safe" exposures for a range of radio and microwave frequencies.

This single safe level has been superseded by the idea of a specific absorption rate (SAR), which describes the amount of energy absorbed in a given time by a given amount (weight) of body tissue. Because the absorption of energy is not the same for different frequencies, the actual exposure level now allowed depends on the frequency of the radio/microwaves in question. The human body has a resonance with electromagnetic waves that are the same length as the human body (around 1 to 2 meters). This means that more energy can be absorbed from exposures to waves of this length. Accordingly, allowable exposure levels have been lowered for this resonance region of electromagnetic waves.[17]

There continues to be a major difference between Eastern European and Western exposure guidelines for radio and microwave fields, with variations of up to a factor of 1000 in the stated limits. For example, a 1989 USSR limit for the general population in the resonance region was approximately 0.02 W/m^2.[18] In contrast, a limit commonly used in North America allows 10.0 W/m^2 for controlled and 2.0 W/m^2 for uncontrolled environments. This marked difference results from a variation in what effects should be considered when setting guidelines.

There are different explanations for these vast differences in safety levels. Some scientists suggest that Russian scientists have used pulsed microwave data, while American scientists have used continuous wave (non-pulsed) microwave experiments to form the basis of their guidelines.[19] Russian scientists have observed central nervous system effects at lower levels than confirmed by American studies. Such effects include depression, memory impairment and inability to make decisions.

Martino Grandolfo, an Italian scientist, attributes the differences between Western and Eastern European standards to different approaches to industrial hygiene. The Eastern European approach defines the maximum allowable exposure as that which does not produce any deviation from the normal physiological state. Their standards are based on the absence or presence of biological effects, and the standards are set without considering the practical ability to reach such levels. Regardless of the allowable level determined, the Eastern European approach is to set the optimum value and goal as zero.[19]

In Western countries various organizations, including government bodies, have used different approaches in the creation of standards.[19] A standard can imply both regulations as well as guidelines that attempt to promote the safety of workers or members of the public. According to Grandolfo, an absolute assurance of safety is often not possible, and the setting of a safety standard depends on the level of risk that is considered acceptable "scientifically and socially." Here again we can see that once risks from technologies are discovered, decisions about the management of these risks involve values and hence, in a democratic society, should have strong public involvement. It is clear that different approaches should be expected between countries and even from different authoritative organizations within a country, and that important decisions which directly affect us should not be left to the "experts".

Public Protection From Electromagnetic Fields

While there is a growing interest in public policy actions that will protect the public from weak fields, the many outstanding problems in understanding the relationship between electromagnetic fields and human health continue to make it difficult to enact such measures.

An example of such difficulty is given in the 1992 Washington State Task Force report on electric and magnetic field reduction.[14] The Task Force report, specifically addressing power line fields, points out that if the voltage level of transmission lines is limited by public policy, this may actually have the effect of increasing magnetic fields in the case where a fixed amount of electricity is to be supplied. This is because a lower voltage necessitates higher currents to deliver the same amount of electricity, and higher currents mean stronger magnetic fields.

Another approach to lowering field exposures would be to increase the number of transmission lines used to carry the electrical power. This would lower the current in each line, and the magnetic fields will be reduced. However, this could increase the number of people actually exposed to fields, albeit lower ones. At this point we don't know which of these situations has the greater impact on public health.

Notwithstanding these kinds of difficulties, the effort to enact public protection measures has begun. Let us begin with an example from Sweden. While Swedish authorities have set thermal-based protection standards for occupational safety and for the general public that are similar to North American guidelines, the Swedish government, characteristically sensitive to public concerns, has taken a prudent approach to the low-frequency magnetic field problem. For example, the Swedish government's National Energy Administration recommended that care be taken not to locate schools, daycare centres and playgrounds near power lines. In a letter circulated in 1990 to Swedish utility officials, the head of the National Energy Administration's electrical safety division suggested that magnetic field levels exceeding 2 to 3 mG should be avoided in such locations, and encouraged caution in new housing developments.[12]

Seven U.S. states have moved to limit public exposure to the electric fields from transmission lines by specifying the allowable electric field level at the edge of the right-of-way. In 1989, the Florida Department of Environmental Regulation created a 150 to 250 mG limit along a power line right-of-way. In 1990, the New York Public Service Commission set a 200 mG magnetic field limit along right-of-ways. The New Jersey Commission of Radiation Protection has considered adopting a similar 200 mG limit, and prohibiting the placement of new children's playgrounds within a right-of-way.[12]

In California and Colorado, public utilities commissions have instructed utilities to practice prudent avoidance and to take "responsible low cost steps to avoid exposing people unnecessarily to these fields."[14] The Washington State Task Force also noted legislation under consideration (but not passed) in other states, including developing strict field limits, delaying new power line construction, and creating a process for looking at field reduction costs and techniques when new lines are being planned. The states involved included Illinois, Washington, Michigan, Massachusetts and Oregon. In Illinois, restrictions on building power lines near schools were included in a bill presented to the legislature.

At the local community level, public exposure to low-frequency fields has been addressed by a number of strategies. For example, the town of Lincolnwood, a Chicago suburb, ordered their local utility to delay construction of a proposed new power line until it can limit magnetic fields to 1.5 mG. In Tennessee, the city of Brentwood set a 4 mG right-of-way limit on magnetic fields and is also requiring that existing power transmission lines be reduced to this level within five years.[14]

In Texas, Florida and California, magnetic fields in school yards have been the focus of concern for school districts. Utilities in some cases have responded with self-imposed field guidelines, or by reducing field exposures by either increasing right-of-way widths or using new designs of lines.

For the most part, public attention has focused on power lines, especially the strikingly visible high-voltage power lines with their ominous metal pylons. Substations and other visible electric equipment have also captured the public eye. To a lesser extent, computers and devices such as waterbed heaters and electric blankets have been highlighted. But the potential for high magnetic fields from household wiring, something which lacks the visibility of a high-voltage line but which can create similar human exposures, has captured less attention. Nor have public radio and microwave sources received the same attention as low-frequency fields from high-voltage power lines.

Static (DC) magnetic fields are only in rare instances encountered by the public. However, that may change. New designs for trains using magnetic levitation techniques demonstrate the potential for technological development to create DC field exposures in the future. The major component of the earth's magnetic field is DC and results in human exposure to a static magnetic field of approximately 500 mG. German researchers are investigating the effects of anomalous local variations in the earth's field on human health and cancer development.[20]

DC transmission lines are, in rare cases, used as an alternative to AC power transmission. Workers in scientific laboratories (especially particle accelerators) and some industrial situations (for example aluminium smelters) are exposed to DC magnetic fields. Guidelines for occupational exposure have been proposed by a number of regulatory bodies.[21] Russian guidelines allow occupational exposures of up to 300 gauss (300,000 mG), and one American scientific laboratory set a limit of 200 gauss for whole-body exposures over an extended period. Other recommended limits are as high as 600 gauss. Workplace exposures to several hundred gauss occur only in specialized industries such as aluminium smelting.

Until recently, radio and microwave safety has been considered in terms of the thermal-based guidelines discussed previously. The idea that there could be non-thermal effects has prompted interest in more stringent standards. Devices such as microwave ovens, cellular telephones and police radar guns all expose people to electromagnetic fields weaker than those required to produce heating (*i.e.*, they meet the thermal-based standards) and thus can be considered "safe" in this respect. The new observations of effects on cells and tissues at levels below this thermal limit raises questions about blanket assumptions of safety from such exposures.

The fact that Eastern European standards were considerably stricter than Western European and North American standards has drawn attention. In California, the Public Utilities Commission is looking into its potential role in mitigating possible health effects from cellular radio-telephone towers.[14] In Seattle, the city and surrounding county have adopted their own limits for public radio and microwave exposures, setting a limit of 200 $\mu W/cm^2$ in the 30 to 300 MHz range. *Microwave News* reported that the Seattle politicians involved in the creation of the tougher guidelines felt that the new limits did not necessarily ensure safety but, they hoped, lowered the health risks. The Seattle city council continues to review new scientific studies on radio/microwave health effects.

The organizations responsible for setting thermal-based radio/microwave protection standards have begun to consider the observations of biological effects at lower levels than previously thought possible. For example, both the American National Standards Institute (ANSI) and the National Council on Radiation Protection and Measurements have created committees to evaluate experiments like those on the calcium efflux effect. Both committees concluded that because they could not directly relate the results of these experimental studies to adverse (or otherwise) human health effects, they could not impact on the present radio/microwave guidelines.[17]

Swedish Computer (VDT) Guidelines

Computers are now being used widely in the workplace in Sweden as elsewhere, and concerns have been raised over possible health effects from the various types of electromagnetic fields emitted by computer video display terminals (VDTs). These nonionizing fields are below the thermal level and are thus safe as far as the thermal standards are concerned. In the effort to specifically address concerns over computer electromagnetic fields, the Swedish government directed the Swedish National Board for Measurement and Testing (MPR is the Swedish acronym) to create a procedure for testing VDTs for electromagnetic emissions. Other health and safety factors including consideration of visual ergonomics are part of the Swedish guidelines, although only electromagnetic fields are of interest here.

The first task was to standardize testing procedures; the electromagnetic fields created by the electronics of a VDT are quite complex, and it is difficult to compare or discuss emission levels without reference to a particular methodology and equipment design for measurements. The second task was to recommend levels for the various fields evaluated by the method. These levels were not based on research of health effects (since Swedish authorities felt that specific risks are still not clearly defined), but rather on what levels were technically achievable by manufacturers.

The first set of test methods, known as MPR-I, were introduced in February 1987, along with recommended field levels. In 1991 a revised set of rules, called MPR-II, were established to deal with several shortcomings in the MPR-I standards. The MPR-II reduced the number of characteristics tested, and simplified many of the testing procedures. Alternating electric fields were added and a new range of low-frequency magnetic fields expanded the previous magnetic measurements. Low-frequency magnetic fields were not considered in MPR-I because concerns over ELF fields were just developing when it was created.

The Swedish rules for assessing VDT electromagnetic emissions simplify the complexity of these fields by using measurements of five different field types and frequency bands. Static electric fields (electrostatic potential), alternating electric fields, and alternating magnetic fields are addressed as part of the MPR-II. In order to accommodate the wide range of electromagnetic frequencies produced by VDTs, the (alternating) electric and magnetic fields are broken into two distinct ranges (5 to 2,000 Hz and 2,000 to 400,000 Hz) which roughly correspond to ELF and VLF.[23] Detailed restrictions on the laboratory testing environment and equipment design are also elaborated in the MPR-II rules.

While many major manufacturers of computer displays have endorsed the Swedish guidelines, there is by no means a consensus on the limits in Sweden. For example, a major Swedish union, the Swedish Confederation of Professional Employees, asked for more stringent limits and test protocols. However, MPR responded to this request by saying that their guidelines are not based on health risks, rather on what is technically feasible to measure and can be currently achieved by manufacturers.

Guidelines like the MPR-II have a number of consequences.

They set a precedent for addressing concerns over workplace exposures to electromagnetic fields, and they set down clear rules for the interpretation and comparison of computer VDT electromagnetic emissions. Such guidelines also exert pressure on manufacturers to reduce the electromagnetic fields produced by the computer workstations they design and build.

MAJOR STUDIES NOW UNDERWAY

There is currently a worldwide research effort into health effects and mitigation, with the number of such studies reaching into the hundreds. Many large and expensive epidemiological studies are underway. The major focus of this effort is on low-frequency fields, especially the magnetic component, produced by electric power systems. Several of these studies are funded by the Electric Power Research Institute (EPRI). They include occupational and residential studies. A childhood leukemia investigation is to be completed in 1994. This study is being carried out at the Cancer Control Agency of British Columbia and is funded by the EPRI, the Canadian Electrical Association, and Health and Welfare Canada. Another study investigating acute lymphocytic leukemia is funded and undertaken by researchers from the National Cancer Institute in the United States. This study, too, is to be finished by 1994. France has launched a leukemia study to be completed in 1994, and in Finland, a study investigating childhood cancers is soon to be published.

In the United States, one of the largest funders of low-frequency field research has been the Department of Energy. In 1992, research was funded in the amount of $7.5 million. There is an effort to create a national program for low-frequency field research in the United States, with funding from both government and industry of at least $6 million annually. Dr. Granger Morgan, a risk management expert working at Carnegie Mellon University, feels that too little research has been done and has recommended federal funding of at least $20 million annually.

Occupational studies currently under way, such as a Brazilian cancer study and a Swedish leukemia study, will contribute their results to the already existing database and will help to guide policies directed at protecting the public.[11,24] However, even such so-called mega-projects can be expected to raise as many questions as answers, and definitive standards and guidelines should not be expected in the near future. In any case, standards and guidelines do not refer to absolute safety. Instead, they are meant to bring risks to acceptable levels, and defining "acceptable" is really a social and political process of many years' duration.

ELECTROMAGNETIC FIELD JOURNALISM

For over a decade, a small independent newsletter called *Microwave News* has collected and published information on technical and public events related to the health effects of non-ionizing electromagnetic fields. The editor and publisher of this newsletter, Dr. Louis Slesin, whose doctoral work at the Massachusetts Institute of Technology concerned environmental risk analysis, has had an intimate insight into the controversy and progress of the environmental electromagnetic field issue. *Time* magazine has characterized Slesin's journalism as "meticulously researched and thoroughly documented."[25] Slesin's editorials have provided a watchdog perspective; several examples will conclude this chapter.

In a 1989 article published in *Technology Review*, Slesin commented on the confusion in dealing with non-ionizing energy in the United States.[26] He pointed out that the job of overseeing and regulating these fields is dispersed among at least fifteen governmental bodies. The Federal Communications Commission regulates TV, cordless and cellular phones; the Food and Drug Administration regulates computer terminal screens, and the Department of Defence oversees its communications and radar network. Slesin suggested there is little cooperation between these various agencies, and that the EPA and National Institute of Health (NIH) should develop a coordinated research effort. In Slesin's words:

> *Until EPA and the National Institute of Health start treating the [non-ionizing electromagnetic] spectrum as a whole, industry and the public can expect more controversy, further development of a crazy quilt of local regulations and still more delays in siting new transmitters and power lines.*[26]

In a 1991 *Microwave News* commentary, Slesin criticized the amount of money and effort being spent on reviewing the literature and setting agendas for future research.[27] He commented that while reviews are being re-reviewed and limited resources are spent duplicating attempts to define future research requirements, no money is being allocated for actual research. Slesin added:

> *In controversial areas of environmental policy, decision makers put off the hard choices by asking for more research. In the EMF business, even this tactic is seen as too risky. Instead they ask for reviews and agendas. This kind of cowardice explains why some of the most interesting work in the field has been supported out of researchers' own pockets . . . it is time to stop stalling and get some work done.*[27]

CHAPTER 5 NOTES

1. Coghlan, A. (1992) "Swedish Studies Pinpoint Power Line Cancer Link." *New Scientist* October 31.

2. Morgan, M.G. (1993) "Risk Analysis Management." *Scientific American* July.

3. Ahlbom, A., E.N. Albert, A.C. Fraser-Smith, A.J. Grodzinski, A.T. Marron, A.O. Martin, M.A. Persinger, M.L. Shelansky and E.R. Wolpow (1987) "Biological Effects of Power Line Fields." New York State Power Lines Project. *Scientific Advisory Panel Final Report.*

4. Carpenter, D.O. (1987) Letter of Introduction to the New York State Power Lines Project. State of New York Department of Health.

5. *The British Columbia Utilities Commission on ELF Health Effects.* July 11, 1989.

6. The commissioner noted that Marino's evidence ensured that all views on this matter were presented to the inquiry but that the costs of hiring Marino were high. An application by the residents' group for the commission to pay for the cost of bringing Marino to Vancouver Island was denied on technical grounds.

7. *Electromagnetics News* (1990) 1:3, 1:4, 1:6.

8. *Microwave News* (1991) 11:5.

9. A letter from the Non-ionizing Electric and Magnetic Field Subcommittee of the Radiation Advisory Committee to the EPA regarding the EPA draft report "Evaluation of the Potential Carcinogenicity of Electromagnetic Fields."

10. This statement echoes a major theme of this book: namely, seeing non-thermal effects in a broader context. Exclusive concern over power line fields in particular shows a lack of understanding of the many other sources of low-frequency fields and the simultaneous controversy over the non-thermal effects of other non-ionizing radiations such as radio and microwaves.

11. Hazan, E. (1991) "EMF Dangerous?" In *Transmission and Distribution* June.

12. *Microwave News* (1990) 10:4.

13. Ferris, H.C., and K.D Simpson (1991) "Delta Phase Configuration To Lower EMF on PacifiCorp's 500 kV Line." *Transmission and Distribution* June.

14. Electric Transmission Research Needs Task Force (1992) "Electric and Magnetic Field Reduction: Research Needs." Olympia: Washington State Department of Health.

15. This is actually an oversimplification since a three-phase line has three conductors, each at 120 degrees out-of-phase from the other; but the idea is similar.

16. Bierbaum, P.J., and J.M. Peters, eds. (1991) *Proceedings of the Scientific Workshop on the Health Effects of Electric and Magnetic Fields on Workers*, held by the National Institute of Occupational Safety and Health in Cincinnati. NIOSH Publication No. 91-111.

17. Petersen, R.C. (1991) "Radiofrequency/Microwave Protection Guides." *Health Physics* 61:1, 59-67.

18. Remember from Chapter 3 that the exact relationship between the electric and magnetic components of these waves means that the allowable levels can be described by the power per unit area, without spe-

cific reference to the magnetic and electric fields. In this case, watts (energy per unit time) represents the power and square meters the area.

19. Franceschetti, G., O.P. Gandhi, and M. Grandolfo, eds. (1989) *Electromagnetic Biointeraction: Mechanisms, Safety Standards, Protection Guides.* New York: Plenum Press.

20. Smith, C.O. and S. Best (1989) *Electromagnetic Man.* New York: St. Martin's Press.

21. Polk, C. and E. Postow (1986) *CRC Handbook of Biological Effects of Electromagnetic Fields.* Florida: CRC Press.

22. *Microwave News* (1992) 12:1.

23. Allowed values are: *(i)* +/- 500 V equivalent surface potential for electrostatic potential, with measurements taken at 0.1 m from the screen surface; *(ii)* 25 V/m for the ELF electric field measured in front of the VDT at a distance of 50 cm; *(iii)* 2.5 V/m for VLF electric field measured at the front, back and sides of a VDT at a distance of 50 cm; *(iv)* 2.5 mG for the ELF magnetic field and *(v)* 0.25 mG for the VLF magnetic field, both measurements taken at 48 defined points around the VDT including 50 cm in front of the unit.

24. Electric Power Research Institute (1990) "Electric and Magnetic Field Research: A Reprint." *EPRI Journal* January/February.

25. *Time* (1990) July 30.

26. *Technology Review* (1989) January.

27. *Microwave News* (1991) 11:6.

SIX

PERSONAL SOLUTIONS

The question of whether weak electromagnetic energy fields can affect living things continues to be answered by more and more observations in the affirmative, and the search for an explanation of how weak fields are able to create these effects goes on. Yet while scientific debate over these issues remains heated, it is the emotional drama of epidemiology that is capturing headlines. Indeed, the main focus of the present research effort is the relationship between weak electromagnetic fields and human health. In Chapter 3, we reviewed our current understanding of weak-field human health effects.

Taken as a whole, cellular, animal and epidemiological studies provide strong evidence that electromagnetic fields can affect human health. But many questions remain. It is a common misconception to view science as being able to provide answers to complex questions in one or several studies, and important questions remain despite hundreds of studies. People need to know exactly what are the risks of living next to a power line? If magnetic fields are the culprit, are the magnetic fields from high-voltage power transmission lines worse or better than the magnetic fields of the same strength from ordinary neighbourhood distribution lines? What should generate more concern — the stronger fields from a hair dryer used over a short period of time, or the weaker fields from power lines over a longer time period? If power line fields are a problem, what about fields from computers or electric blankets? And if diseases like brain cancer take decades to develop, when can assurances be given that newer technologies like cellular phones have minimal risks? Unfortunately there are no answers to these important questions; these are some of the very issues that researchers are addressing.

The U.S. Environmental Protection Agency's internal debate over whether the evidence was strong enough to warrant a "probable human carcinogen" classification for low-frequency magnetic fields is but one example of the level of concern over this issue. Chapter 5 described some of the public dimensions; this chapter will discuss the issue on a personal level.

A basic dilemma emerges as never-before-imagined risks from electrical and electromagnetic technologies present themselves. After a century, electricity is an essential part of our lives and a mythology of progress is so prevalent that we imagine the development of new technologies of this kind as vital for our future. Clearly, then, it is the question of learning to live with the risks of electromagnetic technology, and of striking a balance between risks and benefits, that industrial societies of all political persuasions have had to deal with. How can we enjoy all the benefits of these technologies while minimizing the risks? Deciding what level of risk is considered acceptable involves societal values and political elements that are now being played out.

At the individual level, these basic questions of risk versus benefit, and of how to minimize risks, can also be addressed. Many people try to improve municipal water with filter systems or use purified water sources. Other individuals purchase organically grown food to minimize their risk from pesticides and chemical additives. These individuals are not happy with the generally accepted risks that have emerged in consideration of the benefits from — in these examples — municipal water systems and modern agricultural techniques. The question of risks from electromagnetic fields presents other difficulties. Risks are not yet clearly defined and the definition of what should be considered an acceptable risk is now being dealt with by society. And importantly to the concerned individual, the limitations of electromagnetic field and health knowledge are such that it is difficult to know what are the most effective steps to help minimize personal risks — is it more effective to stop using a hair dryer and electric shaver than to move from a home close to a magnetic field-generating power line?

A strategy known as "prudent avoidance" has been developed to help deal with these difficulties in individual response. As questions about risks from the different types of electromagnetic technologies remain, the most effective approach an individual can take is to evaluate all the ways in which he or she encounters fields of all types, and to take the many simple actions possible to reduce exposure to these fields — in other words, to lower the overall exposure to fields while still being able to enjoy the benefits of electrical and electromagnetic technologies.

This chapter will discuss the origins of the notion of "prudent avoidance" and present some of the ways in which individuals can act to reduce their overall exposure.

PRUDENT AVOIDANCE

A report by Dr. Granger Morgan and other researchers in the Department of Engineering and Public Policy at Carnegie Mellon University, completed in 1989 for the U.S. Congressional Office of Technology Assessment, helped to create a strategy compatible with the desire of many individuals for action while taking into account the many unanswered questions that remain. Morgan's team accepted the mass of evidence that low-frequency fields do in fact interact with cells and organs and can produce biological changes, but that the impact on public health from the fields could not yet be precisely defined.[1] The Carnegie Mellon researchers proposed a policy they termed "prudent avoidance" as a way to approach the problem.

Morgan's concept of "prudent avoidance" is that it is prudent for people to avoid fields, but because of the many uncertainties involved, this should only be applied, at both individual and public levels, if it can be done at modest costs. There are several features implicit in Morgan's statement. Firstly, the fact is that actions to limit risks from technologies are not undertaken until the costs of doing so can be calculated along with the actual benefits of these actions. Secondly, the fact is that the information we need to know whether a particular action is beneficial is just not available, because of our poor understanding of the way in which fields affect us. To cite a specific example from Chapter 5, lowering electric fields actually increases the magnetic field exposure when a given amount of power is transmitted, and early attempts to keep electric fields to a minimum may have only increased public exposure to the magnetic fields that are now the focus of concern.

Morgan has tried to clarify his idea of prudence with an analogy to the dietary choices people are facing as health researchers learn more about the relationship of certain foods and human disease. He prudently tries to cut down on char-broiled meat, and increases his consumption of broccoli, cauliflower and fibre; while not certain that this will protect him from cancer, the available evidence indicates this strategy will reduce the risk. However, he says that he would not rent a refrigerator truck to carry broccoli with him to places where it is not available, and he does sometimes allow his children to eat char-broiled hamburgers. Morgan feels that these kinds of decisions are often made in our private lives but are difficult in a public arena. This is because in many public policy situations grey areas are unacceptable; things are expected to be black and white.

Morgan again reflects a fundamental dilemma we face in our relationship to our technological world. All technologies have some risks that we must bear in relation to their benefits; yet we expect that we can place technologies in two bins — safe or hazardous. The designation of safe that we are so accustomed to hides the reality of risk inherent in all technologies and the fact that someone, somewhere has decided that the risks are small in relation to the benefits. Our doctors tell us medical X-rays are safe, not because there are no risks of cancer associated with this technology but because it has been decided that the benefits far outweigh the risks.

Other researchers have echoed a similar perspective on prudent avoidance. Carl Blackman, for example, suggests a prudent avoidance strategy is one that helps to reduce exposures while taking into account the cost of reduction measures and the current limitations in our understanding of health effects.[2] And at a 1991 conference on field effects in the workplace, held by the National Institute of Occupational Safety and Health (NIOSH), a panel representing the scientists in attendance stated that remaining scientific questions "should not preclude implementing exposure reduction strategies that are now available and feasible."[3]

Prudent avoidance was also discussed by B.C. Utilities Commission chairman John McIntyre in his Vancouver Island power line report. McIntyre stressed that power line fields are part of a broader issue related to the use of electricity, and reiterated the prudent avoidance strategies espoused by the Carnegie Mellon report. McIntyre suggested prudent avoidance could be extended to include limiting the time young children spend playing in power line right-of-ways. Since magnetic fields decrease with distance, in many instances it is easy to reduce exposure simply by putting more distance between yourself and magnetic field sources.

In some instances, power utilities are implementing prudent avoidance strategies themselves, and providing information to the public in this regard. For example, a booklet entitled *Your Guide to Understanding EMF*, used by some utilities, reiterates that as research continues, public agencies and individuals can take actions to mitigate low-frequency field exposure. This means reducing exposures when this can be easily done at little cost. *Your Guide to Understanding EMF* comments on the difficulty in setting health-based standards in the absence of a better understanding of low-frequency field health effects, and that in the absence of such standards, it is up to each of us to consider the potential risks of power frequency field exposures and to decide upon a response.[4]

Your Guide to Understanding EMF describes ways in which you can reduce exposures. These tactics include increasing your distance from electric or microwave ovens when in use, staying back from the TV when it is on, and using hair dryers less. Keeping clocks away from your bedside and turning off electric blankets before going to bed are other suggested measures. Basically, its recommendation is to pay attention to your use of electrical appliances and the fields they produce. In the workplace, for example, the booklet suggests people can sit back from their computer monitor, and recommends arranging work stations in such a way that nobody works within arm's length of the sides or backs of adjacent monitors.

It is important to set concerns about low-frequency field exposures in the context of risks from other sources. *Your Guide to Understanding EMF* points out that people are more inclined to accept risks if they are incurred as a result of their own decisions. Using an automobile, for example, represents a significant risk that most of us choose to incur almost every day; despite the number of deaths and injuries they cause, automobile use is not decreasing.[5]

Individuals have no direct control over the electromagnetic fields produced by power lines, and this may explain the strong emotions they excite. One specific public concern is the epidemiological connection of childhood leukemia to power line magnetic fields. This disease normally affects about one in every 10,000 children. The Feychting-Ahlbom study of power line magnetic fields and childhood cancer, the most powerful of a series of studies spanning more than a decade, found that children exposed to fields over 3 mG had almost four times the risk of leukemia.

Dr. David O. Carpenter, the executive secretary of the New York State Power Lines Project, has also commented on questions of risk.[6] Carpenter points out that media attention has focused almost entirely on the power line question, yet the research carried out for the New York State Power Lines Project suggests that all sources of electromagnetic fields need to be considered. Toasters and electric blankets are examples of other common sources of low-frequency fields mentioned by Carpenter. He noted the Savitz study showed that fields above 2.5 mG may indicate heightened risks, and that many common household appliances often create fields higher than this.

Dr. Robert Becker, in his book *Cross Currents*, also points to the misconception that power lines should be the main focus of concern. Becker, a medical doctor and pioneer bioelectromagnetics researcher, stated that it is not logical to be strongly opposed to a new power line while every night making use of an electric blanket, a device which also results in exposures to low-frequency electric and magnetic fields.[7] It is not hard to understand the focus on power lines, in particular the high-voltage transmission line with its threatening look: these lines invade our communities and we are conditioned to seeing them as dangerous. Electric hair dryers and curling irons, on the other hand, are intimate parts of our daily lives and invoke familiarity, not fear. The strategy of prudent avoidance means recognizing all the sources of fields in our daily lives and taking the many simple and inexpensive steps possible to keep our exposures to a minimum. While research has been strongly focused on power-frequency magnetic fields from power lines, we would be wise to broaden our focus to the other sources of these same fields, whether electric blankets or electric shavers, and to sources of other electromagnetic frequencies such as cellular telephones and microwave ovens.

Prudent avoidance is becoming an established approach to the environmental low-frequency field issue. Exactly what this means in terms of public policy measures is now being worked out in many areas. On the personal level, some individuals, for example smokers, may feel that they have more pressing health concerns than electromagnetic fields,[8] while others, already conscious of the impact of various environmental factors on their health and well-being, may be interested in learning what simple steps they can take to reduce electromagnetic field exposures while still enjoying the benefits of electromagnetic technology.

DO-IT-YOURSELF TESTING

Ideally, a book such as this one would provide you with specific information about the fields in your home. Unfortunately, our experience has taught us that fields are hard to predict. Sometimes you find average fields in a home in the neighbourhood of a scary-looking overhead power line; other times, wiring configurations within walls produce fields in the home that cannot be foreseen. If you want to know about the fields you encounter around your home, you have to take measurements.

Sometimes your local utility might be willing to take these measurements. There's a growing number of private companies that will, for a fee, also provide this service. One such company, operating out of Waterloo, Ontario, is ELMAG Research — run by the authors. If you want to do it yourself — and it's very easy to do — health magazines now commonly carry advertisements for consumer models of measuring devices costing as little as $60, and it is even becoming possible to rent such equipment. In fact, some hobbyists are making their own meters, since all it takes is a coil and an amplifier to sense low-frequency magnetic fields.

If you are interested in the do-it-yourself approach, here are some things to consider in selecting a meter. First, it helps to understand that environmental fields are quite complex and we don't know yet which features of fields relate to health. Therefore, there are different approaches to instrument design, and two different meters may give slightly different readings. This is really not of great concern, as electromagnetic fields from power lines will vary over a day as consumer demand changes. General comparisons of fields in terms of high, average or low are perhaps more useful right now than precise measures. A meter can show how close to a source a person has to be to experience higher-than-average fields, and at what distance from the source fields are reduced to the typical background levels. Thus, there is a lot of useful information to be obtained without scientific precision.

For the most part, you will be interested in low-frequency fields (60 Hz) from power lines, household wiring and all the electrical devices served by our electrical distribution system. Radio and microwaves require more expensive and complex equipment. It is generally the low-frequency magnetic field, not the electric field, that is the focus of concern. Most environmental field meters only measure 60 Hz magnetic fields, but this is not strictly true. One manufacturer offers an inexpensive meter that can respond to radio/microwaves as well as electric and magnetic fields, though with limitations in accuracy. Inexpensive measuring instruments are also available for very low-frequency (VLF) fields of the kind produced by computer VDTs and televisions.

Perhaps one useful recommendation, as far as magnetic field measurements are concerned, is to purchase a meter with three coils. Magnetic fields point in a particular direction, so if a single coil is used, the meter or sensor has to be turned in the magnetic field to achieve a maximum reading (which will occur when the plane of the coil is perpendicular to the direction of the field). This can prove to be confusing and inconvenient.[9] This directional information can be useful for technical personnel (to track down sources of fields for example), but it is unnecessary for most people who do not want to get into the complexity of the magnetic fields. If three coils are used, then the correct reading (or an adequate approximation) is obtained without having to turn the instrument or sensor around, making the measurement process easier.

There is now an effort by the U.S. Environmental Protection

Agency (EPA) to evaluate low-frequency field instrumentation, create standard procedures for measurements, and to help create field reduction strategies. The EPA notes that low-frequency magnetic field exposures from electrical power equipment has been implicated as a public health risk and that many instruments are now commercially available to the public for surveys of environmental fields. The EPA has recently carried out thorough laboratory tests of many of these low-frequency magnetic field instruments, and published its findings in a report that is available to the public. Their test results found a wide variation in the way in which the instruments were designed to respond to the low-frequency magnetic fields.[10]

If you do have a meter that can record microwave measurements, remember that your hand or body can shield these waves. Since it is not likely you would be able to find radio or microwave sources above the thermal limits, a meter sensitive to fields below this level would be of most use. The first place you'll want to take microwave readings is around your microwave oven. As these get older, they tend to leak more microwaves into the surrounding area. Radio/microwave sources also include cordless and cellular telephones and amateur radio transmitters.

If you are able to measure low-frequency electric fields, you will find higher-than-average electric field readings near TVs, computer VDTs, fluorescent lights and high-voltage transmission lines. Your hand can shield electric fields, so the meter should be held between yourself and the source (professionals often mount the meter onto a stick to hold it away from their body).

Again, most environmental electromagnetic field meters will measure low-frequency magnetic fields, with a focus on the power frequency (60 Hz). Power frequency magnetic fields (60 Hz) often occur with harmonic frequencies (120 Hz, 180 Hz, 240 Hz, etc). Meters from various manufacturers will treat these harmonic frequencies differently. Some only measure 60 Hz; others measure a range of frequencies, which will include common harmonics, and add them together according to the actual strengths of each; still others have a so-called frequency-weighted response, giving more importance to higher frequencies.

An example will help illustrate these differences, since some confusion exists about this design question. Consider a field source which has a 60 Hz component of 6 mG and a 180 Hz component of 1 mG measured at a particular distance from the source. A meter with a "60 Hz only" response will read 6 mG; a "flat" response reads 6 mG + 1 mG = 7 mG while a "frequency weighted" response would read 6 mG + (3 x 1 mG) = 9 mG. While the "flat" response is arguably preferable, it is still not clear how to relate health effects to low-frequency magnetic field measurements. Until future research clarifies how a field has to be measured with relation to the health impact, even the right frequency response remains open for interpretation.

These technical points have been presented to help the reader understand more about environmental electromagnetic and radio/microwave fields and how they are measured. Despite these technical details, the actual measuring process is as simple as pushing a button and watching your readings change as you move closer to and away from sources of fields. Meters are widely advertised in health magazines, and appropriate community groups tell you where to find one. If you cannot obtain a information on where to buy or rent a meter, write to us at ELMAG Research, Suite 11 - 421 Barrie Place, Waterloo, Ont. N2L 3Z6.

HOW TO DO YOUR OWN TESTING

This section assumes that you have a meter that can measure low-frequency (60 Hz) magnetic fields. There are three types of fields that are of interest.

The first kind found in the home is the ambient (background) field due to power lines (including high-voltage transmission lines and primary or secondary lines) and substation transformers. Sometimes you can identify the likely source of an ambient field just by looking around for power lines, or a transformer. Take a field measurement at the point on your property closest to the source. Now walk directly away from the source. If the magnetic field reading decreases as you walk away from the source, and does not change as you walk parallel to the source, this would indicate that the dominant background field is from the source in question. If there are several obvious sources, you might be able to identify the most important one by trying this procedure with each source. It may be that several equally significant field sources are present. If readings outside and inside the house are similar, especially when all appliances are turned off, it is likely that fields from neighbourhood sources such as power lines are the most important fields inside the home.

Let us use an example to illustrate the process. Say you find fields of 1.0 mG near a power line, which slowly fall off to 0.5 mG on the opposite side of the property; the home is located roughly in the centre of the property. If fields inside the home range from 0.8 mG to 0.6 mG, with the highest field reading obtained in that part of the home located nearest to the power line, the background field level in the home is determined by the outside source — the power line.

If magnetic fields in the home do not seem to be related to an outside source, you will want to determine their source within your home. One source of fields inside your home is the hidden electrical wiring in the walls, floors and ceilings, especially close to the fuse or junction box, which is where you find the connection to your community's power distribution system. These wires may produce local regions of higher-than-average magnetic fields. If you discover higher-than-average magnetic fields, one prudent avoidance strategy is to relocate beds or seating. Most of these wiring fields do not extend very far from the source.

Your household wiring can create high fields in a number of ways. Older wiring where the wires are not set out in pairs is one example. The phenomenon of ground return current travelling through the plumbing system is another possible cause. Plumbing currents can be affected by neighbours' homes, since the common plumbing network is often used to ground domestic electrical systems. There are other ways in which higher-than-average wiring fields can be produced in the home, all of which are related to unequal currents in the paired wiring.

Another possible magnetic field source is ceiling cable electric heating. This is not too hard to track down since these fields will change from floor to ceiling level, and they will cycle on and off according to the thermostatic control. This type of electrical heating is not commonly used and you will be aware of its presence in your home.

The identification and reduction of wiring fields is now beginning to be studied. This whole area is new, and firm answers are not readily available. It may be difficult to track down the exact cause of higher-than-average wiring fields, and even more difficult to correct the problem. New devices are coming to the market to help with plumbing-related problems. Rewiring can be the solution. In some cases only a small change may be required; in other cases, more extensive changes might be required to bring about improvement. This information is meant to suggest the nature of the solutions; do-it-yourself electrical changes are discouraged. The reduction of wiring fields via electrical changes means that risks of electric shock and fire hazards have to be considered. If you have a problem with wiring fields, contact your local utility or an electrician.

After testing for background sources and in-house wiring fields, you will want to measure the third type of field source: low-frequency household electromagnetic devices such as toasters, hair dryers, televisions, microwave ovens and electric stoves. The first thing you will want to note is how great the field is close to the device. Next, observe how far away you have to get before the fields drop to background levels. You can use this information, together with the knowledge of how far away you typically are when using the device, to create strategies for reducing exposure. Moving your bedside electric clock farther away from your bed or turning off your waterbed heater before retiring are examples of personal prudent avoidance strategies.

MAKING SENSE OF THE FIELDS

Once you have measured the low-frequency magnetic fields in your home, you will be interested in making sense of the reading. If you do not have your own meter, you may have had measurements taken by a company that specializes in this area, or by a representative of your local utility. There is at this time no clear level against which your readings can be compared. One approach is to compare the fields in your home to other homes. The following values are suggested by us:

< 0.2 mG	Below average field
0.2 to 1.0 mG	Typical field
1.0 to 3.0 mG	Slightly higher than average field
> 3.0 mG	Higher than average field

Dr. David Carpenter, director of the New York State Power Lines Project, has suggested guidelines for making sense of the average fields measured in your home. He based these guidelines on an epidemiological study of childhood leukemia by Dr. David Savitz. Given the uncertainty in the epidemiological results, he cautions that these represent rough guidelines only.[6] Carpenter's guidelines for average ambient fields:

< 1.5 mG	Lower risk
1.5 to 2.5 mG	Some risk
> 2.5 mG	Higher risk

These guidelines are supported by the Feychting-Ahlbom results. These Swedish researchers completed the most powerful study to date of the risks of living close to high-voltage transmission lines. When they divided children into three categories depending on the fields they experienced from transmission lines near their homes, they found a relationship between childhood leukemia risk and the average magnetic field strength as follows:

< 1 mG	Normal risk
1 mG to 3 mG	Relative risk of 1.5
> 3 mG	Relative risk of 3.8

Be careful to note that these are *average* fields measured throughout your home. It is normal to find some areas of your home with higher-than-average readings.

If you discover higher-than-average readings in your home, you may want to discuss this with a power utility representative. Some utilities will take measurements for you with professional equipment to verify the readings that you have obtained with your meter.

PRUDENT SOLUTIONS AND NEW PRODUCTS

There are presently no standards or guidelines set down by authorities to use as a guide. As the science and politics surrounding the creation of standards continue, it becomes a matter of personal motivation to evaluate risk-versus-benefit questions and to make decisions to practice prudent avoidance. The many remaining unanswered questions mean we don't know yet what the most effective prudent actions might be. For example, it is not possible to evaluate the differences in the impact on our health between brief exposures to high magnetic fields from a hair dryer and continuous exposure to lower fields from power lines. The best approach is to consider all possible field sources and to take what you feel are reasonable actions to limit exposures — the strategy of prudent avoidance.

The best course to take will become clearer once you've combined an awareness of your use of electrical devices with an understanding of the way in which the fields behave. Keep in mind that much of the present focus of concern is on the low-frequency (60 Hz) magnetic field. The following sections provide some basic considerations for prudent action and a discussion of relevant products.

Ambient Fields

If you live in a neighbourhood where higher-than-average ambient fields are present, one prudent avoidance recommendation is to restrict children's play in higher-field areas. Monitor Industries, a company based in Boulder, Colorado, has developed a room shield that could be used in a living room or bedroom to lower higher-than-average background fields. This device is an active field-cancelling system. This means that the field in a living room or bedroom is measured and an equal and opposite field is created to effectively cancel out the room field. Such a device is fairly expensive and is only useful in certain situations.

Wiring Fields

There are instances where the most significant magnetic fields will be created by household wiring. Such concerns can be approached by clearly identifying the cause of the fields. As discussed in the section on testing, possible causes of higher-than-average fields from household wiring are now being investigated. If older styles of wiring are the cause, rewiring with carefully paired wires will correct the problem, although this is expensive. Sometimes minor changes in wire configuration at electrical panels or outlets can solve the problem.

Higher-than-average fields related to using the plumbing system as an electrical ground can be reduced in a number of ways. For example, you can insert a special piece of pipe (a non-conductive barrier) into the buried water line outside your foundation. This piece will prevent currents from flowing through the plumbing system on their way back to the neighbourhood power line. Eliminating a plumbing current may help to reduce unbalanced currents and hence lower magnetic fields in your home.

Unfortunately these kinds of changes are expensive too, and altering the grounding of a home's electrical system should be approached with caution. If grounding efficiency is reduced, shock and fire risks may increase. One company has developed a ground connector which automatically reestablishes grounding to the water main if a serious electrical fault develops. According to the company, a large number of high fields in homes could be reduced by eliminating plumbing currents.

Again, we recommend against changing your electrical wiring without professional assistance, especially that of a qualified electrician. Electrical wiring, specifically grounding techniques, have evolved to effectively prevent electrical shock and fire hazards and should not be changed without careful consideration and the help of someone who knows what they are doing. Most electricians are not yet familiar with techniques for reducing magnetic fields, so finding appropriate professional assistance may be difficult. (One of the only sources of information at this time is Monitor Industries, 6112 Fourmile Canyon, Boulder, Co. 80302.) Again, you can avoid areas of higher-than-average magnetic fields by simply moving a bed or sofa.

Computer and Television Electromagnetic Fields

There is increasing interest in reducing the electromagnetic fields produced by computers, in particular the cathode ray tube style of video display terminal (VDT). Because VDTs presently in use do not have any problems with the high-frequency waves known as X-rays, it doesn't help to wear lead aprons — a practice that is still being carried out in some workplaces. Occupational health authorities feel that these devices may create undue back strain and may exert pressure on the fetus.[11] Despite the common misconception to the contrary, lead is not useful as a shield for low-frequency magnetic fields.

A consideration of VDT electromagnetic fields can be incorporated into purchasing decisions. The New York City school system, for example, follows a policy of prudent avoidance, and uses standards based on the Swedish MPR-II guidelines when evaluating computers for purchase. The New York standards are even more stringent than the Swedish recommendations.[12] The school system has found that lower-field models cost about the same as the ones which emit higher magnetic fields.

In 1991, Air Canada replaced the terminals it used in its airline operations after tests showed that old equipment didn't meet the Swedish guidelines. They were replaced with units that met the guidelines.[13]

It may be difficult to obtain information about the electromagnetic fields from different computer models, since few salespeople are knowledgeable about this issue. A recent informal survey of sales personnel confirmed this paucity of accurate information.[12] In some cases companies are reluctant to provide this information. For example, one Apple Computers spokeswoman stated that they do not publish emission numbers for their computers because they do not believe computer fields pose a health risk.[14] Despite this, the careful consumer will find many computer monitors that are advertised as meeting the MPR-II guidelines.

Sitting back as far as comfortably possible is an effective way to prudently reduce VDT fields. Since field levels can be larger at the back and sides of the VDT, care can be taken in the placement of adjacent units in a crowded office setting. Low-frequency magnetic fields will penetrate walls and room dividers.

Attachable shields, which reduce electric and electrostatic fields, are also available for video terminals. These shields have conductive coatings and also function as anti-glare screens. Anti-static screens should not be confused with anti-glare screens that do not have electric field reduction capability. One way to tell them apart is that a screen that reduces electric fields will have a grounding wire. These screens are available in glass and less expensive mesh versions, and while they reduce the electric and electrostatic fields, they have no effect on magnetic fields.

Low-frequency magnetic fields are a focus of concern, and they are notoriously difficult to shield. Several products are available to reduce the magnetic fields from VDTs, as a number of companies are competing to provide solutions to magnetic field concerns. One company offers a service where they will insert mu metal shielding to reduce magnetic fields. Mu metal is a special alloy that helps to trap the fields in the source. Mu metal boxes and strips are also being marketed for magnetic field reduction. These products are relatively new additions to the computer accessory marketplace.

Television electromagnetic fields are similar to those created by a computer monitor. The difference is that people watching television sit much farther back than computer users. Sitting as far back as comfortable, and preventing children from sitting too close to the set, are prudent avoidance tips.

Your TV produces electromagnetic fields and consumes electricity even when it's not on, so you might decide to unplug it when you're not watching. Magnetic fields extend in all directions from the television, and penetrate walls. If you have your own meter, measurements of fields could be incorporated into purchase decisions. (We're not aware of any North American model currently on the North American market that is advertised as low-field.) The anti-static screens used to reduce computer electric fields could also be used for a television.

An interesting product recently developed for the German market is an "environmentally friendly" television. Whenever possible, the Ökovision uses recyclable tin, aluminum, and solid wood instead of plastic and presswood in its construction; any plastic that is used is clearly marked for easy sorting during recycling. No lacquers are used to put it together — only screws and "safe" glues. The packaging the Ökovision comes in is made from natural materials, and is supposed to be returned to the manufacturer for reuse.

Although the effort has been made to create a recyclable unit, the Ökovision is advertised to produce electromagnetic fields below the Swedish guidelines. The fields from this television are stated to be several thousand times less than those produced by a typical television.[15]

Prudent Avoidance Around the Home

Simple steps can be taken to reduce exposure to electromagnetic fields from electric blankets and waterbed heaters. For instance, you can heat up your waterbed during the day and turn the heater off while you're sleeping, instead of the other way around. Similarly, an electric blanket can be used to heat up the bed and unplugged before bedtime.

Although fluorescent lights can be more economical than incandescent bulbs, they produce larger low-frequency fields. Identify fluorescent lights that are within arm's length of where you spend a lot of time — desk lamps, for example. If you use a space heater, keep it in a remote corner of the room. Fields from motor-driven electric clocks and telephone answering machines can be avoided by keeping them away from your bed. Consider using battery-powered or wind-up clocks instead.

Try standing back when you're using an electric stove or microwave oven. Use the back burner of an electric stove instead of the front burner. Older microwave ovens will leak more microwaves through old door seals than a newer unit; you might want to have an older microwave oven tested regularly. Try to locate it in a low-traffic area of the kitchen.

Hair dryers and electric razors create strong fields, though they are not used for long periods of time. You could consider restricting their use as much as possible, or replacing the electric razor with a blade (and get a closer, smoother shave in the bargain!).

Electromagnetic Devices for Health Promotion

While some authorities are recommending prudent avoidance of electromagnetic fields, new devices are appearing that claim to use magnetic fields to improve medical conditions such as circulatory problems and chronic pain. Other devices, ranging from pendants and plates to special watches, are promoted to "override electromagnetic pollution."

Scientific evidence does demonstrate that electromagnetic fields can have an effect at cellular levels, and both negative and positive effects on human health have been reported. However, present scientific understanding precludes an accurate prediction of either positive or negative outcomes from exposure to a particular type of electromagnetic field. As a result, the use of any such devices should be approached with a critical eye.

CHAPTER 6 NOTES

1. Morgan, M. Granger (1991) "EMF Dangerous: Expert Opinion." *Transmission and Distribution* June, 15-28.

2. Blackman, C.F. (1991) "Do Electromagnetic Fields Pose Health Problems?" *Frontier Perspectives* 2:2, 11-16.

3. Bierbaum, P.J., and J.M. Peters, eds. (1991) *Proceedings of the Scientific Workshop on the Health Effects of Electric and Magnetic Fields on Workers*, held by the National Institute of Occupational Safety and Health in Cincinnati. NIOSH Publication No. 91-111.

4. Culver Company (1991) *Your Guide to Understanding EMF (Electric and Magnetic Fields)*. Public information brochure used by utilities.

5. Fries, J.F. and L.M. Crapo (1981) *Vitality and Aging: Implications of the Rectangular Curve*. New York: W.H. Freeman and Company.

6. Carpenter, D.O. (1987) Letter that introduces *The New York State Power Lines Project Report*.

7. Becker. R.O. (1990) *Cross Currents: The Promise of Electromedicine, the Perils of Electropollution*. Los Angeles: Jeremy P. Tarcher.

8. Cancer risks from smoking are interesting to note. The lung cancer rate in the non-smoking population is 3.4 per 100,000. Smokers of

more than one pack per day face a risk of over 200 per 100,000. Smokers also increase their risk of cancer of the cervix, bladder, kidney, pancreas and stomach 50 to 200 per cent compared to non-smokers.

9. Low-frequency magnetic fields are most commonly sensed with a coil of wire and an amplifier. Manufacturers of instruments with only a single coil often recommend taking three readings in mutually perpendicular directions, squaring each result, adding them together and taking the square root to obtain the correct reading instead of rotating the meter in the field until a maximum reading is obtained.

10. "Laboratory Testing of Commercially Available Power Frequency Magnetic Field Survey Meters." Environmental Protection Agency Report No. 400R-92-010, June 1992.

11. Charron, D. (1988) *Health Hazards of Radiation From Video Display Terminals: Questions and Answers.* Hamilton, Ont.: Canadian Centre for Occupational Health and Safety.

12. *VDT News* (1992) January/February.

13. "Got the VDT's" (1992). In *CAW-TCA Union, the National Magazine of the CAW-Canada* 5:2, 20.

14. "VDT study finds link to miscarriage." Hamilton *Spectator*, December 8, 1992.

15. "Ein Fernsehgerät, das sich gut wiederverwerten lässt." *Natur* 11, 1992.

GLOSSARY

Alternating current (AC) — Alternating currents change direction at regular time intervals. For example, currents in our homes produced by the 60 Hz power system change direction 60 times each second. The fields produced by these currents have corresponding directional changes.

Amplitude modulated (AM) — Waves have both amplitudes and frequencies. As in AM radio, information (lower frequency) is mixed into a radio wave (higher frequency) by modulating its amplitude.

Antigen — An antigen (usually a carbohydrate or protein) is a substance that is foreign to the body and will induce an immune response which produces specific antibodies that link up with the antigen.

Bioeffects — Short for biological effects. Bioeffects refers to changes observed in living things, whether cells in the laboratory or animals and humans. In this book it refers to the biological changes produced by electromagnetic fields.

Bioelectromagnetics — The new branch of science that studies the relationship between electromagnetism and life.

Carcinogenesis — The process of the development of a cancer.

Case-control study — In epidemiological studies, people who are diagnosed with a certain disease ("case") are compared to those who do not have the disease ("control") to help identify those factors that are associated with the disease.

Cellular membrane — The outer boundary of cells, giving cells their structure, form and rigidity. The cellular membrane is semi-permeable, allowing only certain molecules to pass through as nourishment for the cell. Waste products leave the cell through the cellular membrane.

Central nervous system — A system of nerves composed of the brain and spinal cord. It is the control centre of the nervous system and receives sensory input from the peripheral nervous system.

Circadian rhythms — Biological processes that occur in cycles of approximately 24 hours, even when organisms are isolated from their normal environment.

Coherence domain — A region of material in which there exists a coordinated excitation of the quantum states.

Coherent excitation — Introducing energy into a system in a coordinated way. This has implications for biology because of the potential for long-range interactions of molecules.

Confounder — In epidemiological studies, large numbers of people are studied to determine the various factors that are associated with disease. Sometimes an observed positive association between a disease and the particular factor being studied turns out to be false because of some other hidden factor — called a confounder — that the study failed to take into account.

Current — A flow of electric charge in an electrical conductor (wire).

Cyclotron resonance — In this book, a phenomenon known as cyclotron resonance was discussed as a way in which weak electromagnetic fields could influence biological organisms. Cyclotron resonance involves an ion moving in a circular path under the influence of a magnetic field. When a second field is applied with a frequency that matches the ion's circular motion, a resonance condition occurs where a maximum absorption of energy is possible.

Delta configuration — A particular arrangement of the conductors of a power line that is used because it produces electromagnetic fields smaller than conventional arrangements.

Direct current (DC) — Currents that do not change direction are said to be direct. Direct current power systems are seldom used, although solar voltaic homes may use this type of power. Direct currents produce static, unchanging fields.

Distribution lines — These power lines operate at lower voltages than transmission lines and distribute power throughout a community from substations to homes, factories and offices.

DNA (deoxyribonucleic acid) — The primary hereditary molecule, by which genetic material is passed from generation to generation.

Efflux of calcium — Tissues such as brain tissue have calcium ions that are bound to the tissue surface. Electromagnetic fields may trigger the release of the bound calcium ions. This release is called an efflux.

Electric field — An energy field related to the force experienced by an electric charge.

Electromagnetic spectrum — The complete range of oscillation frequencies of electromagnetic waves. Divided into two basic types: ionizing and non-ionizing.

Electromagnetic wave — A wave containing both electric and magnetic fields that are oriented perpendicularly to each other and to the direction of travel. Waves of different frequencies have different physical properties.

ELF (extra low frequency) — The lowest part of the electromagnetic spectrum, usually 3 to 3000 Hz; electromagnetic waves with low frequencies and long wavelengths. Includes the 60 Hz power frequency.

EMDEX (electric and magnetic field digital exposure) — A small portable instrument for measuring electric and magnetic fields. It can be worn by a person and will take measurements at regular intervals over the course of the day.

EMF (electromagnetic field) — A field containing electric and magnetic energy. Although not strictly defined as such, EMF is increasingly used to refer to only energy fields with low frequencies, especially extra low frequency (ELF) magnetic fields.

EMF bioeffects — The changes observed in biological organisms as a result of exposure to weak electromagnetic energy fields.

Enzyme — Proteins that promote biochemical reactions in living organisms.

EPA (Environmental Protection Agency) — A United States governmental organization with responsibilities for environmental matters.

Epidemiology — The study of the relationship between the frequency of disease occurrence and the factors associated with the disease in human populations.

EPRI (Electric Power Research Institute) — An organization funded by electric power utilities that is responsible for carrying out research related to the transmission and distribution of electricity. It has sponsored studies focusing on health effects of electromagnetic fields.

Frequency — The number of complete cycles of a wave that occur in a second. Measured in Hertz (Hz).

Frequency modulated (FM) — As in FM radio, information (lower frequency) is mixed into a radio wave (higher frequency) by modulating its frequency.

Gauss (G) — A commonly used unit of magnetic field measurement, where: 1 G is equal to 1000 mG, 1 G = 10^{-4} Tesla (T), 10,000 G = 1 T.

Harmonic — The power frequency of 60 Hz has harmonic frequencies of 120 Hz, 180 Hz, etc.

Hertz (Hz) — A unit of frequency describing the number of cycles per second.

Hormone — A substance produced in the body in small quantities that is used for regulation in cells or organs.

Immune system — A bodily system that protects against the invasion of foreign bodies (antigens) like bacteria and viruses.

In vitro — Describes experiments using living cells that are carried out in a glass dish or test tube, separate from the organisms from which they came.

In vivo — Describes experiments that are carried out using whole living organisms.

Ion — An atom that has a net positive or negative charge due to a loss or gain of electrons.

Ionizing radiation — Electromagnetic energy with enough strength to dislodge electrons from atoms and molecules and thus able to disrupt the basic biochemical structures of life.

Leukemia — A type of blood disorder where the white blood cells proliferate in an uncontrolled manner. These cells are unable to perform their tasks related to the immune system.

Lymphoma — Cancer of the lymphatic system.

Magnetic field — An energy field created by moving electric charges which can produce forces on other moving charges.

Magnetic organ — An organelle of a magnetite crystal surrounded by a thin membrane. Magnetic organs have been found in organisms as diverse as bacteria, bees, pigeons, salmon and humans.

Melatonin — An important regulatory hormone produced by the pineal gland. Involved in the control of circadian rhythms and regulation of brain activity.

Microwave — The part of the electromagnetic spectrum lying between infrared light and radio waves. These are short waves that have more energy than ELF, VLF, and radio waves.

Modulated — Electromagnetic waves are said to be modulated when their amplitudes or frequencies are varied. This is how FM and AM radio work.

MPR — The Swedish acronym for the Swedish National Board for Measurement and Testing. The Swedes have developed testing procedures and allowable levels for the electric and magnetic fields from computer displays (VDTs).

NIOSH (National Institute of Occupational Safety and Health) — An American governmental organization that has sponsored conferences and research on the relationship between electromagnetic fields and occupational safety and health.

Non-ionizing radiation — Electromagnetic energy without sufficient energy to dislodge electrons from atoms and molecules. This includes microwaves, radio waves, VLF and ELF.

Non-thermal effects — Effects on cells and organisms from non-ionizing electromagnetic energy fields at levels below that required for heating. How these biological changes come about is unclear at the present time.

NYSPLP (New York State Power Lines Project) — After public hearings related to the construction of a new transmission line in New York State, this almost decade-long research project was set up to investigate questions related to health effects from electromagnetic fields. The project was completed in 1987.

Office of Technology Assessment — A U.S. government department that sponsored a report which promoted the idea of prudent avoidance.

Peripheral nervous system — A system of nerves that connect outer parts of the body and its receptors to the central nervous system.

Pineal gland — An outgrowth of the forebrain in the centre of the head. The gland is involved in the production of the hormone melatonin which controls circadian rhythms.

Plumbing current — In many homes, the electrical wiring is connected to the plumbing system. This means that currents may flow through the metallic pipes. These plumbing currents produce magnetic fields.

Power frequency — The frequency at which our electrical systems operate. North America uses 60 Hz electrical systems; Europe uses 50 Hz.

Prospective study — This type of epidemiological study examines a group of people considered free of disease, but exposed to the hypothesized disease-causing factor. This group is followed over time so that the differences in rate of developing the disease can be seen in relation to the exposure factor. The group of people that is followed over time is called a "cohort".

Protein synthesis — The process of making proteins which occurs in all cells. Genes control the structure of the proteins that are manufactured.

Prudent avoidance — More research is required in order to fully understand the relationship between electromagnetic fields and human health. Prudent avoidance is a strategy, recommended by some authorities, that addresses concerns over electromagnetic field exposure while taking into account the importance of electricity in modern life. It suggests that simple steps can effectively reduce overall exposure.

Pulsed — Electromagnetic radiation is said to be pulsed if it is produced with off and on cycles.

Quantum theory — A theory of dynamic systems which hypothesizes that energy exists as small packets (quanta). This revolutionary theory was developed early in this century.

Radio wave — The part of the electromagnetic spectrum lying between the microwave and VLF regions. Radio waves are commonly used for communications.

Resonance — A system which likes to vibrate at a certain frequency will strongly interact with an outside force when that outside force vibrates at the same frequency as the system. This matching of internal (system) and external (force) frequencies is called resonance and when this occurs the force will have the largest effect on the system possible.

Right-of-way — A corridor in which a power line is built, used by the power company during construction and operation of a power line.

RNA (ribonucleic acid) — RNA is closely associated with DNA. Its major function is the manufacture of proteins.

Sinusoidal — Waves can have different forms — square, saw tooth, sinusoidal etc. A sinusoidal wave looks like a smooth up and down ocean swell; named after the sine function of trigonometry which describes its shape.

Substrate — The substance in a chemical reaction that is acted upon by an enzyme.

Thermal effects — Effects on cells and organisms related to the heating ability of non-ionizing electromagnetic energy fields. Microwaves and radio waves have enough energy to produce heating; 60 Hz fields do not.

Thermal noise — The higher the temperature of a material, the more motion the atoms and molecules of the material undergo. This type of random motion is called thermal noise.

Thermodynamics — That branch of physics dealing with the study of heat and its interactions with other forms of energy.

Transformer — Transformers are electric devices used to change the voltage of the incoming power.

Transmission line — A power line operated at high voltages used to carry electrical energy from its site of production to communities where the electrical power is needed.

VDT (video display terminal) — The name given to the television-style monitor used to display information necessary during the operation of a computer. The term "VDT" is often used to refer specifically to cathode ray tube-type (CRT) monitors.

VLF (very low frequency) — The part of the electromagnetic spectrum lying between the lowest frequency region (ELF) and the radio frequency region.

V/m (volts per meter) — A unit of electric field measurement.

Voltage — The work required to move a unit electric charge from one place to another.

Wavelength — The distance between two identical points on a wave in consecutive cycles.

Weak electromagnetic energy fields — The focus of this book. This refers to non-ionizing electromagnetic energy that is too weak to be able to cause heating damage to living systems.

This includes microwave fields like that from a cellular telephone and the 60 Hz fields that surround a hair dryer.

Windows — Weak electromagnetic field bioeffects sometimes only occur within certain ranges of frequencies and intensities, called windows. Increasing or decreasing the frequency or intensity will remove the observed biological changes. There are both frequency and intensity windows.

Wire coding — Instead of using difficult-to-obtain magnetic field measurements, some epidemiological studies have made use of the fact that magnetic fields are closely related to current, and classified or coded power lines according to the amount of current in the line.

INDEX